BEE Fit

Baby Enhanced Exercise Fitness

Dear Sally
and Brodie
I hope Eleanor
enjoys the book
Lots of love
Gemma xx

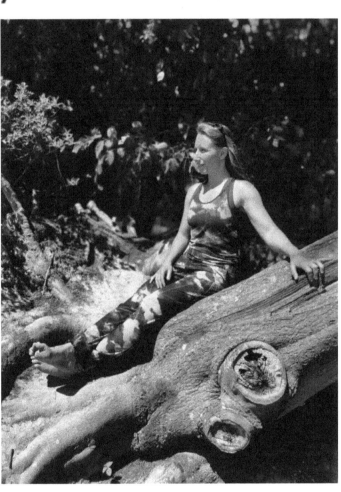

GEMMA NICE

First published in 2020 by Ingram Spark

Gemma Nice has asserted her right under the Copyright, Designs and Patents Act, 1988, to be identified as Author of this work.

A catalogue record for the book is available from The British Library.

Library of Congress Cataloguing-in-publication date has been applied for:

ISBN: Print: 978-1-8382885-0-1

ePub: 978-1-8382885-1-8

ACKNOWLEDGEMENTS: Photographer Jim Browning

Book cover design: Camilla Fellas Arnold

Illustrations: Daisy Dawson

Models: Gemma Nice, Hugo Nice and Brianna Nice

Design: Gemma Nice

Outfits: Sweaty Betty

Buggy: GB Pockit

Baby Wrap: Moby Baby Wrap Carrier

To find out more about our author visit www.easyoga.co.uk. Here you will find extracts, author interviews, details of forthcoming events and the option to sign up to our newsletter.

For Hugo and Brianna, my wonderful children and for my husband Darren. Thank you xxx

Contents

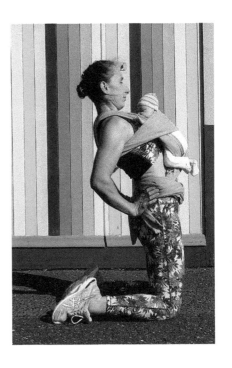

Introduction and about the author

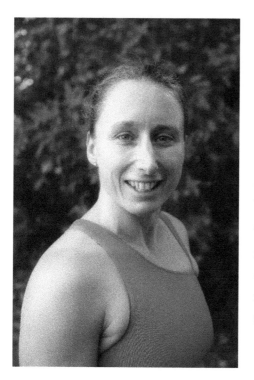

Hello and welcome to this book. My name is Gemma and I've been into sport, yoga, health and wellness for as long as I can remember. As a parent of two, I understand that time to work out or going to the gym is mostly non-existent. This book will give you tips and advice on how to work out using strength training and yoga incorporating your children into your workouts either at home or in the park. This is by means of baby wearing in a wrap/sling or using the buggy.

This book is intended for parents whose babies are more than twelve weeks old. This is due to some of the exercises or yoga poses using the core muscles of the mother and her diastasis recti may not have fully healed yet.

My husband and I used to be in the gym every day before we had children. This obviously couldn't work once they were born so I had to come up with exercises and a yoga practice at home or at the park. It's easy to incorporate this into your daily routine if you have the right mind set and this is where this book comes in if you need the extra help or push. It's an easy to follow guided book with yoga poses and exercises with little motivational quotes on every page to help keep you going.

In 2006 my husband and I went backpacking around the world and while in Thailand I saw people practising Yoga on a deserted sandy beach. It just looked idyllic to me and that's when I became hooked on yoga. I bought an idiots guide to yoga while we were in Malaysia and started practising every day.

I found that it really relaxed and energised me. So, when we got to New Zealand, I bought a yoga mat which I still use today. When we got home after our travels I signed up to yoga classes and haven't looked back since. In August 2013 I qualified as a Hatha yoga teacher with over 200 hours of yoga practice via the home studies group BSY. I wanted to teach other people about the benefits of yoga regarding both body and mind as I'm so passionate about it. I then went on to qualify in Ashtanga Vinyasa Flow yoga which is the basis of my classes now.

Our son was born in January 2014 and then in June 2017 our daughter was born. I was very active during both pregnancies which I think has helped me to lose the baby weight. There is so much stigma around pregnancy and exercising. I always believe you are the only one who knows your body better than anyone else. Take it slow and at your own pace and carry on doing the things you always were doing.

I am not your typical yoga teacher. I do not chant, or 'om' and this book reflects this. I love to connect with my children and my exercising and yoga practice is just built around five or ten minutes when I get a chance every day. They find it normal now that I'm just hand standing around the house or using them as weights for lunges or squats. Our son loves a piggy back when I am working out. It's fun and interesting for them and I think it's healthy that they have active parents. This helps with the interaction and bonds of both parent and child.

I am not a nutritionist but I have an interest in it where I have shared with you in this book. There is also a nutritional plan and a guided four-week plan for you to follow. You can also just pick up and put down the book whenever you need to. There is a guided relaxation and visualisation technique to help you if you are stressed or just need a bit of 'me' time, as well as two breathing techniques. I've also written about Diastasis Recti and New workout motivation.

This book is split into chapters to make it easier for you to follow. Some of the chapters are baby wearing in a wrap and others are using a buggy for the exercises. Some are both baby wearing and using a buggy.

So, use this book how you wish. Keep active and most of all enjoy your workouts with your children.

Gemma xxx Gemma Nice

Disclaimer

You should consult your doctor or other health care professional before reading this or any other fitness book or programme to determine if it is right for your needs. This is particularly true if you (or your family) have a history of high blood pressure or heart disease, or if you have ever experienced chest pain when exercising or have experienced chest pain in the past month when not engaged in physical activity, smoke, have high cholesterol, are obese, or have a bone or joint problem that could be made worse by a change in physical activity. Do not start using this book if your doctor or health care provider advises against it. If you experience faintness, dizziness, pain or shortness of breath at any time while exercising you should stop immediately.

This book is not a substitute for medical attention, examination, diagnosis or treatment. Yoga is not recommended and is not safe under certain medical conditions. By reading this disclaimer you affirm that you alone are responsible to decide whether to practice yoga or take part in the exercises specified within this book. You should knowingly, voluntarily, and expressly agree to accept full responsibility and assume the risk for your use of this book.

This book offers fitness and nutritional information and is designed for educational purposes only. You should not rely on this information as a substitute for, nor does it replace, professional medical advice, diagnosis, or treatment. If you have any concerns or questions about your health, you should always consult with a physician or other health-care professional. Do not disregard, avoid or delay obtaining medical or health related advice from your health-care professional because of something you may have read within this book. The use of any information provided within this book is solely at your own risk.

If you have been advised that your Diastasis Recti has not fully healed then I probably would not recommend to do some of the exercises within this book until you have been fully signed off by your practitioner or health care professional. Go at your own pace and when you feel ready to, use this book as you will. Taking care wherever you need to.

The exercises included in the book are safe to perform and are effective for new mothers postpartum. Please read the above disclaimer for more information. There is no risk for new mothers who are in good health.

Justin Edwards AFAA approved Ante and post-natal Personal Trainer.

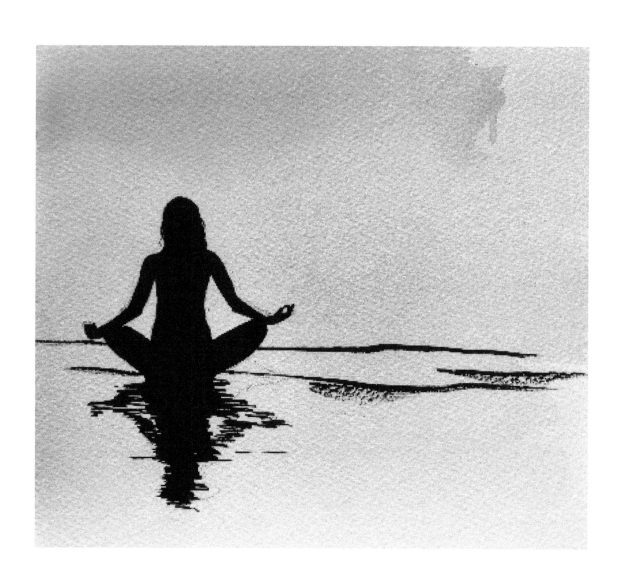

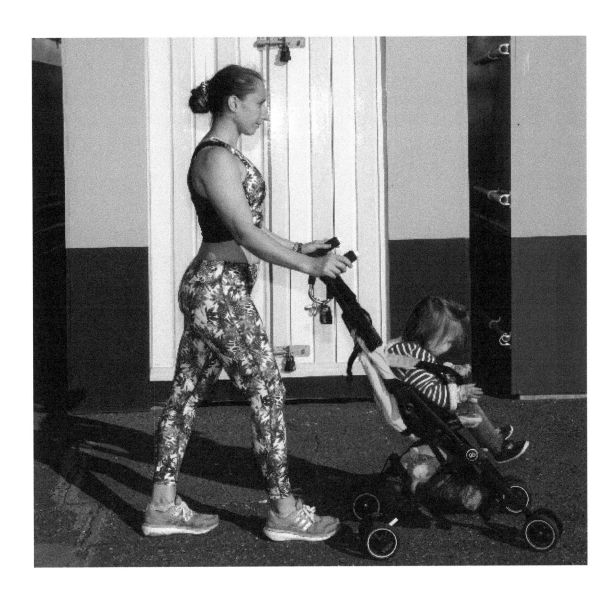

Chapter One

Breathing Techniques

Diastasis Recti

New Workout Motivation

Walking and Running with a buggy

Relaxing Breathing Techniques

There are so many different types of breath techniques. These two I find are the best to fully relax and calm the mind. As parents we need to take five minutes out of our day to just concentrate, bring our mind back into our body and fully connect within ourselves. The two breath techniques described here are Ujjayi Breath and Calming Breath.

Calming Breath

This is great to really allow your body and mind to connect and de-stress.

Method

1. Come to a comfortable seated position having your eyes open or closed, whichever feels more comfortable.

2. Take a few deep breaths here. Inhaling and exhaling through your nostrils.

3. On your next inhale really use the diaphragm and draw the breath right up into the lungs, keeping shoulders down away from the ears. As you inhale slowly count to three.

4. On your exhale, slowly release your breath using your core muscles, counting to four. Try to lengthen the out breath as much as possible. Say to yourself on your inhale 'let' and on your exhale 'go'. Notice the stress and tension release from the body.

5. Repeat this technique for as long as you wish.

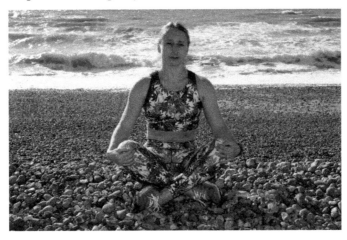

Ujjayi Breath

Ujjayi or translated means 'Victorious' breathing, is a breathing technique which is used to calm the body and mind. It is used in Vinyasa Flow yoga as a means of connecting the poses with the breath. This breath also calms the mind and gets the brain to concentrate on something else if you are stressed at all.

Ujjayi breathing naturally lengthens the breath allowing your lungs to get the extra inhales it needs to fully clam the mind and body.

This breath is also known as 'Ocean Breath' as it sounds like the waves of the ocean. So, put on some comfy clothes, come into a comfy seated position and enjoy breathing.

Method

1. Come to a comfortable seated position having your eyes open or closed, whichever feels more comfortable.

2. Take a few deep breaths here, inhaling and exhaling.

3. Now we're going to try a technique to help you understand how the breath works at the back of the throat. Bring one hand up towards your face with the palm facing towards you. Take a big deep breath in through your nose and when you exhale have your mouth open and blow into the palm of your hand. Imagine you are fogging up a mirror with your breath. You should be able to feel the warmth of the breath on your hand. Do this for three breaths.

4. Now do the above again but this time closing your mouth but still imagining huffing up the mirror on your hand. This will open and close the back of your throat. Try this for a couple of breaths. You will hear a sound like Darth Vader at the back of the throat. It can also sound like the ocean waves - that's why it can sometimes be called 'ocean breath'.

5. Stay here for five or six breaths. Then find your breath's natural rhythm.

Come here wherever you need this breath. It's such a relaxing breath.

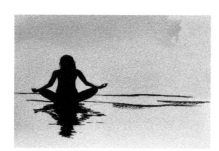

'Deep breaths are like little love notes to your body.'
– Lovethispic.com

Page 12 Relaxation and Breathing

Diastasis Recti

What is Diastasis Recti?

A human being is made up of muscles and bones which all connect to form you. Obviously, you know this from biology class at school. We will now be talking about the 'abs or core' area of the body as this is where you can potentially find Diastasis Recti.

The abdomen is formed of a band of muscles called Rectus abdominis or abs or core, whichever you would prefer to call it. This band of muscles usually have six combined muscles all connected side by side in three pairs. These are the muscles which we talk about when referring to the abs or core or even a 'six pack'.

These muscles have an area down the middle called a Linea Alba or connective tissue. This area has little blood supply to it. This is what knits the muscles together. When a lady becomes pregnant the Linea Alba stays the same for an amount of time, but in the later stages of pregnancy this line then splits in two to give more room to the baby on its expansion. The pregnancy hormone Relaxin also helps with this process. As the name suggests this hormone starts to relax the body getting ready for the birth process. Relaxin stays in the body for around six to eight weeks post-partum.

How can I tell if I have Diastasis Recti?

The more severe your split, the more finger widths you will be able to fit through the gap. Come to a lying down position with your feet flat on the floor and knees bent. Bring one hand up to the area where your navel is. Lift your head off the floor slightly and bring the chin towards your chest so your core is engaged. Press down with your index and middle fingers with your thumb facing towards your chest and the little finger down towards your pelvis. Have your fingers placed just above and in line with your navel. You should be able to feel muscle here. If your fingers feel like they are caving in or the inside of your body, then this is called a diastasis.

The severity of this can range from one finger width to four or five finger width. The latter being classed as severe. Move the fingers down below the navel and check here repeating the same procedure. The abdominal muscles may be split in different areas.

Another way of telling if you have a Diastasis is if your tummy is protruding above your navel. This looks like a bulge or a 'pregnancy tummy' even though you are not. Some people may think you are around six months pregnant and this can lead to an embarrassing conversation for everyone involved. If you have gone back to your pre-pregnancy weight but still have a 'tummy' this may be due to a Diastasis which has not knitted back together by itself.

How can I rectify Diastasis Recti?

Another way of telling if you have a Diastasis is if your tummy is protruding above your navel. This looks like a bulge or a 'pregnancy tummy' even though you are not. Some people may think you are around six months pregnant and this can lead to an embarrassing conversation for everyone involved. If you have gone back to your pre-pregnancy weight but still have a 'tummy' this may be due to a Diastasis which hasn't knitted back together by itself.

You can get back to your pre-pregnancy body if you have Diastasis Recti with more severe gaps needing more work on your core or abs. This will take time so be patient. When you have given birth, it takes your internal body one whole year to get back to normal. So, keeping this in mind, aim for a year to get your core stronger. There are roughly four areas we need to cover here to help you with this. They are: core work, posture, eating right and breathing correctly.

Core work – Find your core and pelvic floor muscles (see 'What is diastasis recti?'). Start to slowly engage your core and pull up the pelvic floor area. See below for more information on some safe exercises. DO NOT do any crunches as these increase the pressure around the muscles and connective tissue and will do more harm than good. The more the connective tissue is stretched, the more it will lose strength and get thinner. This will then make it a lot harder to start again.

Going slow will help you to build up the strength around the areas which need attention.

There is also a cosmetic surgery option to repair the connective tissue but please try to repair them yourselves. I believe in you! You can do this!

Posture – Make sure you have the correct posture. Read Mountain Pose on page 35 for more information. The correct posture will make sure you have less abdominal pressure. Try not to wear high heels as this really puts your whole body out of alignment. Try to wear flat shoes.

Eating right – To help repair the split muscles you need to eat the right foods. You will need collagen boosting foods, for example Vitamin A and Vitamin C, Zinc, Proteins, Iron, Essential fatty acids, and a lot of water. Go to the nutrition section for more information.

Breathe correctly – Make sure you are breathing using your diaphragm and not just the upper part of your lungs. You will need to use the full capacity of the lungs as this will help relieve the pressure. Try to keep your shoulders down and relax. For more information go to the relaxation section of the book which has a few breathing exercises.

Is it Too Late to Correct a Diastasis Recti?

Sometimes the Linea Alba will automatically knit back together after birth once the pregnancy hormones have gone. This can be between three to six months post-partum. Sometimes it can take years, so just be patient and work on it. It will only get better with a little help from you.

There are a few exercises or yoga poses you can do to help strengthen this area. They are:

Bridge pose (see page 97)

Cat/Cow Pose (see page 49)

Wall Sit (see page127)

Standing Side Bends (see page 39)

'I always believed. And when you do that, life can get unbelievable.' Jessica Ennis-Hill

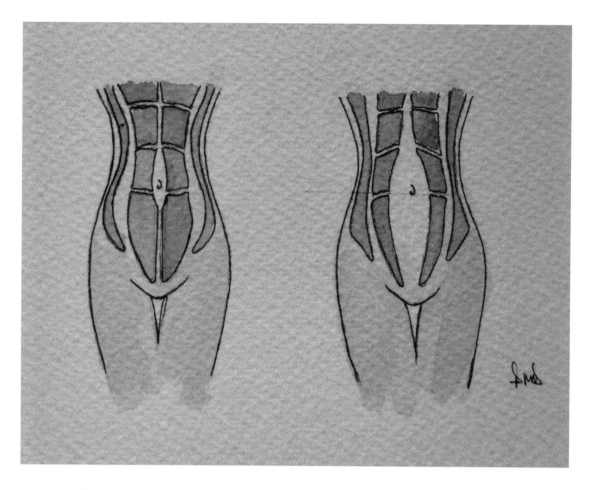

Correct Diastasis Recti   **Not correct Diastasis Recti**

The Pelvic Floor Muscle's

The pelvic floor muscles are a band of muscles which lie across the base of your pelvis. They are there really to hold all the pelvic organs in, the bladder, uterus, and intestines. These muscles are held in place by ligaments which support the pelvic organs. If there is an increase in pressure for example carrying a heavy item, bending, or straining, the ligaments brace so that the internal organs such as the bladder and uterus are not forced downwards. These muscles help to keep the bladder and bowel openings closed to help stop urinary incontinence and will relax to allow urine and faeces pass when needed. They also help with posture in conjunction with using the spine. The pelvic floor muscles may have been stretched during childbirth and the common symptoms you will be finding are:

- Increased involuntary bladder leakage when coughing, sneezing, or laughing.

- Urgency to need the toilet right away.

- Going to the toilet too often.

- Leakage of bowel movement with increased pressure for example lifting to heavy.

- Heaviness in the vaginal region.

- Lack of sensation during sex.

If you are feeling any of these symptoms, then you will need to start exercising your pelvic floor region.

To find your pelvic floor come into a comfortable seated or laying down position. Relax. Squeeze and draw in your anus as if you are holding in wind. Squeeze around your vagina and bladder tube as if you are stopping the flow of urine mid flow. You may feel a tightening of the muscles as you pull up. Do not hold your breath and keep relaxed. Make sure you do not pull in your stomach. Try not to squeeze your glutes and keep your legs relaxed.

Aim to squeeze for ten seconds and then fully relax. Rest for a few seconds, then repeat these squeezes until you feel the muscles get tired. Try to aim to do these for three to four times per day. During some of the exercises and yoga poses in this book, I give reference to engaging your pelvic floor muscles. This means doing this exercise and keep it squeezed until you come out of the pose or you cannot hold it any longer. Engaging your pelvic floor muscles will help to engage your core muscles, strengthening both your core and pelvic floor muscles.

New Workout Clothes Motivation

Whether you are embarking on a new fitness journey or are trying to get your old journey back, you need some motivation. This is where a new set of workout clothes comes in.

Notice how they make you feel. You are aiming to feel alive, energised, motivated and wanting to work out. If you are aiming to lose some or all the extra weight gained through pregnancy, this is a great way to start.

If you have a goal in mind, then keep sight of this. Try to break this goal down into achievable little bite-sized pieces. So, for example if you pushed yourself further one week and achieved more than you were expecting, reward yourself. Maybe buy another piece of gym wear or treat yourself to another motivational piece of equipment. Always reward yourself.

If you fall short of that particular goal, do not give up and don't be hard on yourself as this will set you back. Keep going and do not let the demons in your head tell you otherwise. Of course, the demons will pop up every now and again. This is natural. Keep going. The end is in sight.

'Believe in yourself and you will be unstoppable.'
– Emily Guay

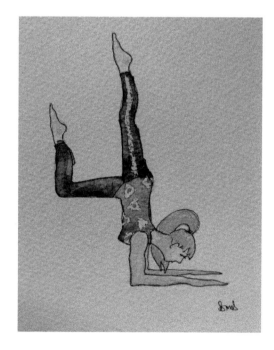

Walking and Running with a buggy

Taking a stroll or a light run will get you out of the house, help with post-natal depression, make your legs stronger and will burn off calories. It will also clear your mind helping you to think straight especially if you are or have been sleep deprived.

Try to get out the house and go for a walk once a day. You will feel so much better for it.

Start off with a small, slow stroll and work up to a faster pace when you are feeling stronger especially in the pelvic floor region.

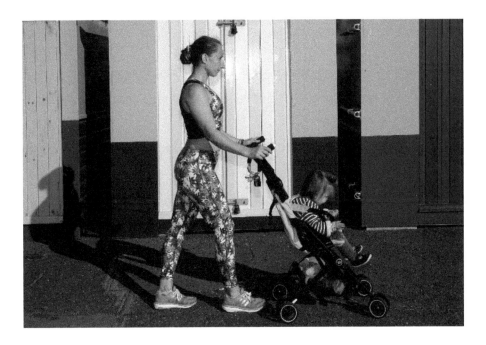

Try a variety of different areas you are most comfortable with as this will make you feel more confident for example a walk around your local park or a walk in the woods. Either have your baby in a buggy or wrap. Having baby in a wrap is so comforting and a great bonding experience for you both.

When thinking about starting up running with the buggy, take it slow. Go to a place which has familiar surroundings, and you know the area well. Start off with a five-minute walk for a warmup then a one-minute jog, back to a one-minute walk and two-minute run doing this for a total of twenty minutes. Try this for three times a week.

When you feel stronger, up the walk/jog/run to one and a half minutes of running, one and a half minutes of walking, three minutes of running and three minutes of walking. Try to do this twice over.

Next would be to split the walking by half and add in a pyramid style training session. For example, run for three minutes then walk for one and a half minutes. Run for five minutes then walk for two and a half minutes. Run for three minutes then walk for one and a half minutes.

As you slowly begin to up the running, add in a small amount of walking to bring your heart rate down to a slower rate. The start to up the running again. Slowly but surely you will start to feel stronger and fitter.

Always make sure you start with a brisk five-minute walk for a warmup. This will increase the blood flow to all the muscles and joints ready for the run.

Pushing a buggy either walking or running will add slight resistance to your normal pace. For running holding the buggy handle, this is slightly harder as you have not got the use of the power in your arms due to them on the handle. Try swapping each hand to push the buggy, keeping the arms loose and not engaged.

Tips

Be careful if you have knee or joint injuries. Also, be aware of your pelvic floor strength. A high impact exercise like running can possibly set you back with the repair of the pelvic floor muscles. Please be careful and go at your own pace. Start slowly and work up. Even if you are a seasoned runner, after giving birth the body has changed significantly and needs time to heal. Your brain may say you are ready to go back to training, but your body may not.

A post-partum body takes up to one year to be back to a pre-pregnancy state. Be kind to your body. Love it, it's just gone through an incredible journey.

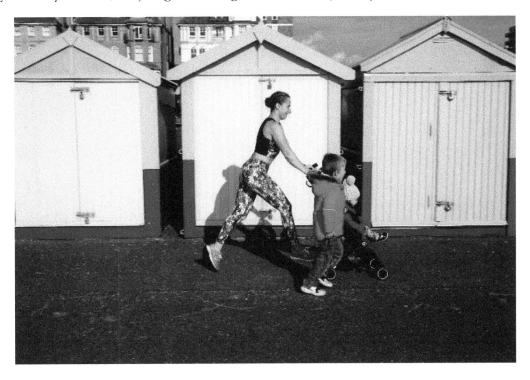

Wake up with determination. Go to bed with satisfaction - Unknown

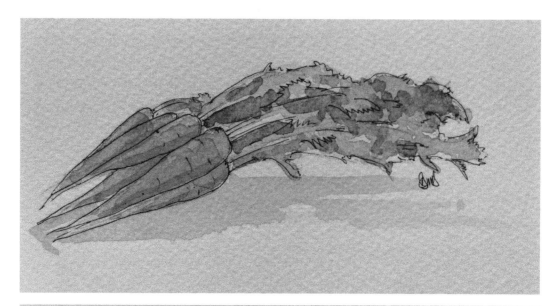

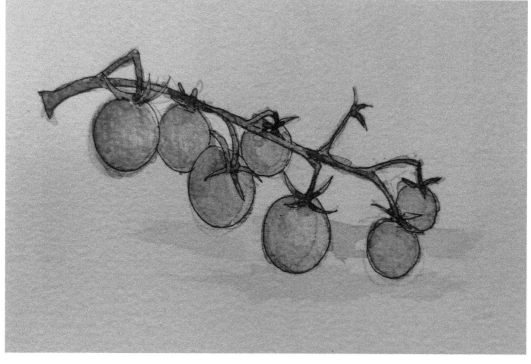

Chapter Two

Nutrition

Nutrition

Nutrition can be a minefield, so it's a good idea to start with the basics.

We need nutrition to keep healthy and stay alive. This means that our bodies do not produce any nutrition, so we need to source this from food and water. Nutrients are vital for disease prevention, growth and good health. These are then broken down into two categories: Macronutrients and Micronutrients.

Macronutrients come in the form of actual large quantities of food and help to provide your body with energy. These are protein, carbohydrates and fat.

Micronutrients come in the form of vitamins and minerals which are only needed in small amounts.

Carbohydrates

Carbohydrates are the energy blocks from your food. They contain good sugars which help to fuel your body for everyday activities. They help with brain function and the main central nervous system (sending nerves throughout your body). Carbohydrates can also help protect against diseases such as cancer.

Sources of Carbohydrates

Not all carbohydrates are good ones. You are aiming to go for non-processed types with no refined sugars, for example, wholemeal bread, whole-wheat pasta, noodles, and rice. These are better than the white varieties as they will not lead to a spike in blood sugar concentration (insulin spike). Whole-wheat foods release this sugar (and, therefore, insulin) slowly, so your body has time to use it in the correct way. Also, aim to eat beans and fibre rich vegetables, including carrots, beets, broccoli, artichokes, and sweet potatoes.

Fibre is a type of carbohydrate that the body can't digest. Though most carbohydrates are broken down into sugar, fibre cannot be broken down into sugar, and instead it passes through the body undigested. fibre helps regulate the body's use of sugars, helping to keep hunger and blood sugar in check.

Different fruits have high fibre content in them. For example, apples, bananas, oranges, strawberries, and some exotic fruits. All these are a great source of good fibre.

Fats

Fats usually get quite a bad rap, but they are an essential part of a healthy diet. Healthy fats help with the absorption of vitamins and minerals, help to build cells, help with movement of muscles and are a great energy source. Healthy fats can also help with balancing blood sugar levels and improve brain function, helping to reduce the risk of Alzheimer's disease. They also help in the production of Testosterone. Testosterone will not make you bulk out, it helps to regulate the hormones. But also a high fat and high sugar diet will be detrimental to your testosterone levels especially in men. In women testosterone plays a role in reproduction, growth and general health.

Sources of Fats

Unsaturated fats are great for the body. They provide essential fatty acids that your body cannot synthesise itself. Saturated fats should be limited as these can have the reverse effect on the body by eating to much saturated fat can lead to high blood cholesterol. This can clog up our arteries and restrict the blood supply to our heart which in turn may cause a heart attack.

The most commonly known unsaturated fats are omega 3s and omega 6s. These are mostly found in nuts, seeds, oily fish (e.g. salmon), oils such as avocado, flax seeds and olives. Another amazing oil is coconut oil as this is plant-based so has a faster uptake by the organs to use as fuel to the body.

Saturated fats come in the form of animal-based sources, for example butter, cheese and red meat, processed meats including sausages, mincemeat, animal skin, bacon and fatty cuts of meat. Limit your intake of these to reduce heart disease. For example, a small matchbox size piece of cheese once a day.

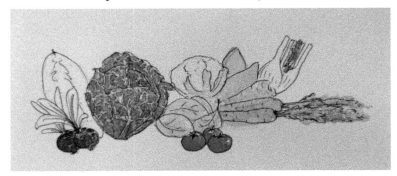

Protein

Protein is amazing for muscle repair, not just for gym bunnies but in everyday life. It is part of every cell, every tissue and organ in the body. It also helps to produce hormones. Protein helps with the building of antibodies to help prevent and fight disease.

Proteins come in the form of amino acids and the body needs 20 of them to stay healthy. They are then broken down into essential amino acids and non-essential amino acids. There are nine essential amino acids which are not made in the body so need to be found in the form of food. There are 11 non-essential amino acids which are made by the body.

Each protein is constantly being broken down. The body does not store proteins like it does other nutrients, so this needs to be given to the body in the form of food every day. Therefore, most of your portion control should be based around protein as the body needs it to repair and grow constantly. Most of the protein we need to fuel and repair our bodies comes in the form of high-quality protein. This mostly comes from animal or plant-based sources. It is hard to find the balance of obtaining protein sources that aren't high in fats and carbs. For example, a handful of nuts contain a high fat content but also are very good for you. Plant based diets are harder to find protein in. Some examples are mentioned below.

Sources of Proteins

Lean white meat is a good place to start, for example chicken or turkey.

Fish, including salmon, haddock, and bass - any type of fish.

Dairy products, for example eggs, milk, cheese, and yoghurt.

Plant-based food such as tofu, nuts, beans, and pulses.

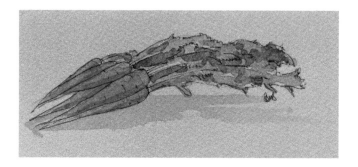

Vitamins and Minerals

Vitamins

Vitamins and minerals are needed to help keep the body functioning correctly. They help to fight off any diseases and repair bones and tissues. They heal wounds and help boost the immune system. They can also help to repair cells and convert food into energy.

Vitamins can be split up into two groups. They are water soluble and fat-soluble vitamins.

Water soluble vitamins are found in all types of foods. They are absorbed into the blood stream and help the body to release energy, to build energy, to help repair broken cells, and make collagen which helps to repair wounds and forms a base for teeth and bones to be built upon. Water soluble vitamins are Bs and C.

Fat-soluble vitamins help to keep your eyes, skin and lungs all in good condition. They help to build bones and protect the body with antioxidants.

Fat-soluble vitamins are A, D, E and K. They can be found in fatty foods and oils. Fruit and vegetables are a good source of vitamins and minerals and should come from a wide range. You should try to eat over a third of your daily intake in food per day. It is recommended that you eat at least 5 portions of fruit and veg per day. This can include fresh, frozen, juiced, canned or dried.

Minerals

Minerals help with the daily function of the body. They help to build strong bones and teeth (calcium) as well as build hair, skin and cells. They also help with metabolism in the body.

There are several major minerals the body needs to function daily. They are: calcium, zinc, iron, fluoride, chloride, magnesium, phosphorus, potassium, sodium and sulphur. Some of these help keep the water balance right as most of our body is made up of water (around 60%).

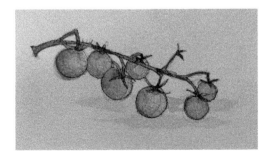

You will source most of these vitamins and minerals from a healthy balanced diet through eating five or more portions of fruit and veg per day.

Water

Water is probably one of the most important nutrients you need for your body to function correctly. We are made up more of water more than anything else. Water will help ward off dehydration. It helps to improve your overall mood and helps with brain function. It helps to carry nutrients around in the bloodstream faster and carries more nutrients to all the cells. It also helps with the digestive system and keeps the intestines flowing by preventing constipation.

We should aim to drink around two to three litres of water each day to keep the body functioning at its best. Water does not just have to come from a tap. It can be found in fruits and vegetables such as watermelon, cucumber, or spinach. It is a good idea to drink around one pint of water when you first get up in the morning and then around one pint just before bed. This will kick-start the kidneys and urinary tract to wake up and function well. You can tell your hydration state by the colour of your urine. If it's very yellow and has a strong smell, then you are dehydrated. If it is a faded yellow colour and not smelling, then you are perfectly hydrated. This is what you are aiming for.

Here is a list of a few foods to eat. These will give you all your nutrition for your daily requirements.

- Greek yoghurt, natural yoghurt
- Small matchbox size cheese
- Cottage cheese
- Butter
- Whole Milk, almond milk, coconut milk
- Eggs
- Lentils
- Quinoa
- Meat (lean white meat e.g. chicken, red meat in small amounts)
- Fish (tuna, salmon, white fish)

- Spinach
- Green beans
- Peas
- Beetroot
- Pomegranate
- Broccoli
- Courgette
- Carrots
- Lemon
- Avocado
- Chilli
- Ginger
- Sweet Potato
- Pepper
- Broccoli
- Kale
- Onion
- Tomatoes
- Mushrooms
- Aubergine
- Whole wheat pasta, whole wheat rice, whole wheat spaghetti, noodles, freekeh
- Good quality granola
- Nut butter, for example peanut butter, almond butter, cashew butter
- Coconut oil
- Water, green tea, herbal teas

- Butternut squash
- Corn on the cob
- Bananas
- Peaches/nectarines
- Kiwi
- Cherries
- Melon
- Strawberries
- Pears
- Natural nuts not flavoured or salted (pure cashews, peanuts, almonds)
- Seeds (Chia seeds, Flax seeds)
- Dried fruit
- Hummus
- Cucumber
- Olives
- Tofu
- Rye bread, sourdough bread
- Pesto
- Protein shake
- Good quality dark chocolate 70% or more

Breakfast, Lunch, Dinner and Snacks

I've devised a few meal plans. Feel free to add or takeaway anything. You need to make sure you are eating roughly every three hours. This is to accommodate your blood sugar levels to stay at a constant level. For example, if you eat at 7.30am, try and eat around 10.30-11.00am which would be a snack. Then lunch, a snack in the afternoon and then dinner.

Breakfast

- Scrambled eggs, poached eggs, omelette
- Greek yoghurt with fresh fruit and honey
- Good quality granola, yoghurt, fresh fruit
- Porridge with honey, fresh fruit and seeds
- Fresh fruit and vegetable smoothies with chia seeds
- Protein powder smoothie
- Soaked overnight oats with seeds, berries, and fruit
- Smoothie bowl
- Protein pancakes with honey and fresh fruit

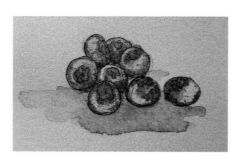

Snacks

- Hummus with carrot sticks
- Protein shake
- Feta cheese
- Hard boiled eggs
- Small handful of nuts and raisins
- Carrot sticks
- Greek yoghurt
- Three squares of good quality dark chocolate (70% or more cocoa)
- Olives
- Fruit
- Rice cakes
- Homemade oat cookies
- Homemade granola bar
- Homemade protein bars

- Apple with nut butter

Lunch

- Baked sweet potato with small amount of butter, with either tuna mayo, hardboiled egg, chicken, or feta cheese
- Salads with two hardboiled eggs, whole chicken breast, feta cheese with olives such as a Greek salad, chicken pesto, or chicken quinoa and rice salad
- Tuna pasta, chicken pasta
- Quinoa burger
- Salmon curry
- Stir fry
- Turkey and avocado sandwich
- Yoghurt
- Fruit
- Small amount of good quality dark chocolate
- Tofu and avocado sandwich

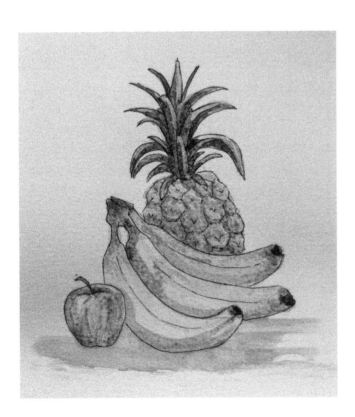

Dinner

- Stir fry with lots of vegetables and lean meat or tofu
- Spelt or cauliflower rice pizza
- Sweet potato lentil bowls
- Tuna whole wheat pasta bake
- Teriyaki glazed chicken salad
- Baked salmon fillets with vegetables

- Kale Caesar salad
- Tuna steaks
- Chicken burrito bowls
- Roast chicken or turkey
- Cod, lentil and broccoli

- Homemade salmon fish cakes and vegetables

- Mediterranean chicken

- Chicken or turkey whole wheat pasta with feta cheese sauce

- Homemade Thai chicken curry
- Pork chops with loads of veg
- Homemade chicken or turkey pie with veg
- Homemade burgers grilled and not fried
- Meatballs

Processed Foods or Refined High Sugar Foods

This is a huge subject, but we will just concentrate on the basics.

Sugars will be hidden in most foods which tend to be processed. There are different processing procedures in the food industry. We all know which foods are good for us and which are bad. For example, crisps, biscuits, varieties of chocolate, sweets, cakes etc. The list is endless. We should only eat these foods in moderation. Sugars can also be hidden on the ingredients list, for example named as sucrose and fructose.

If a food has been through a process to get to its final product, then it can be bad for you. You are aiming for it to be as unprocessed as possible. For example, milk, whole milk is better for you than skimmed as it's gone through less processes to get to its final product state. Just use your common sense for most of the foods you eat. Processed food can also contain harmful substances like carcinogens which may bring on cancer. Putting different chemicals into foods will help them to have a longer shelf life and to taste better. These can be harmful to our bodies. If you are not sure on a certain ingredient, then do not buy it.

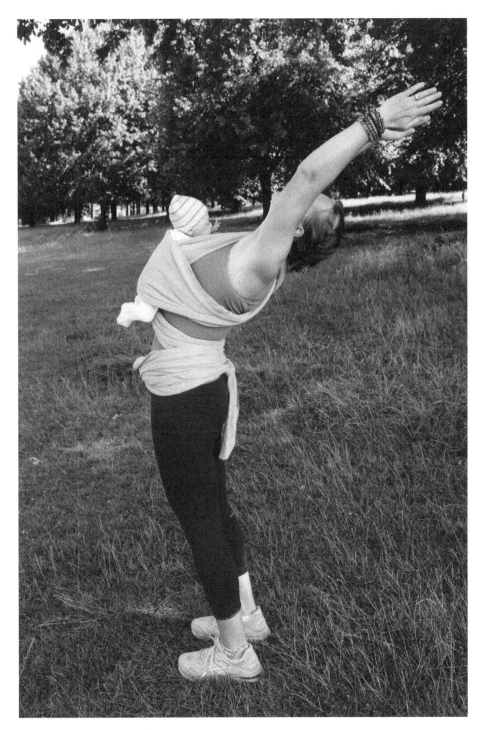

Figure 1 - Example of a Back Bend

Chapter Three

Warm up exercises and yoga poses baby wearing or baby in a buggy.

These exercises can be used to relax as well as used as a warmup or cool down.

Mountain Pose

Standing Side Bends and Back Bends

Head and Neck Stretch

Cat and Cow Pose

Butterfly Pose

Cow Face Arms

Half Forward Fold Buggy Pushouts

Mountain Pose

The benefits of this pose are amazing. It improves posture, allows you to feel grounded, improves stability and confidence. It is used as the basis for all the standing poses and if you are tired during your exercise you can come back into Mountain Pose at any time. Enjoy.

Being a parent can be incredibly stressful at times. Mountain pose is great to just stand and take a few deep breaths in and out, releasing tension and stress all over your body.

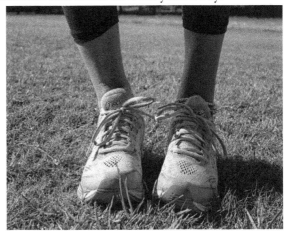

Method

1. Stand with the bases of your big toes touching heels slightly apart. Slowly and gently lift and spread your toes and the balls of your feet, then lay them softly down on the floor. Make sure all five toes are on the floor spread out evenly.

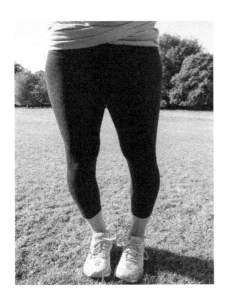

2. Slowly lock your kneecaps into your thighs and then lift the inner ankles to strengthen the inner calf muscles. Turn the upper thighs slightly inward. Lengthen your tailbone toward the floor and lift the pubis toward the navel. You are trying to get your whole body in a straight line all the way from the tips of your toes to the crown of your head.

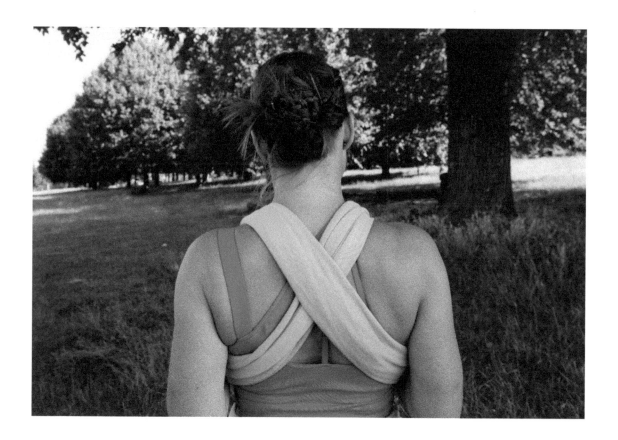

3. Press your shoulder blades into your back, then widen them across and release them down your back keeping them away from your ears.

4. Make sure that the crown of your head is directly over the centre of your pelvis, with the underside of your chin parallel to the floor.

Let your arms hang
down beside your
torso. You can also
have them in prayer
position just in front
of your chest.

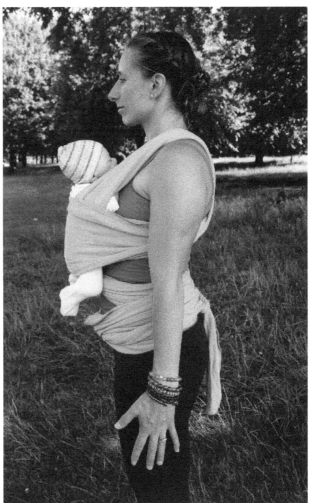

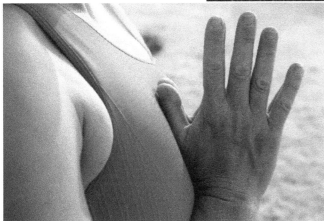

5. Stand here in Mountain Pose and breathe. Big deep breaths. Eyes open or closed, which ever feels comfortable for you.

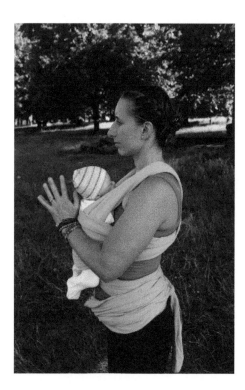 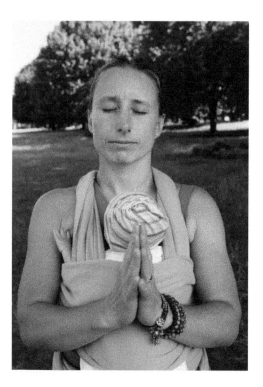

If you are feeling stressed then come into Mountain Pose and stand here for 10 minutes or so, just deep in breaths and deep out breaths. At the end of mountain pose, take an inhale and exhale 3 times, with the exhale being a sigh sound. This will release any tension left in your body.

Tip

Be careful when doing Mountain pose if you suffer with Headaches and low blood pressure.

Close your eyes and imagine the best version of you possible. That's who you really are. Let go of any part of you that doesn't believe it. – C.Assad

Standing Side Bends and Back Bends

Side bends and Back bends increase the flexibility in your spine. This is a great pose to do if you are breast feeding as your posture is all out if you are feeding in an awkward position. This is also nice if you have lower back issues due to carrying baby around.

Other benefits include releasing tension and stress in your body, especially around the neck and shoulders. It corrects your posture and massages your internal organs. It also stretches your spinal nerves and muscles. It allows the lungs to expand so you have fuller deeper breaths allowing more oxygen to flow around your blood stream. It really energises the body so if you are feeling sluggish due to lack of sleep give this a go.

You can either have your baby in a wrap attached to you or have him/her in the buggy next to you.

Back Bend Method

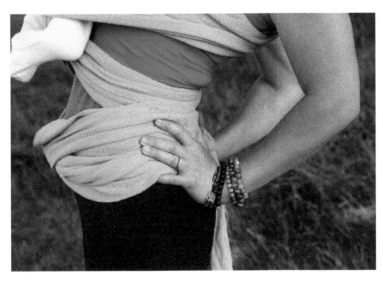

1. Stand in Mountain Pose (turn to page 35 for instructions for Mountain pose) and bring your hands to wrap around your waist with fingers pointing towards your pelvis. Bend backwards slightly so there is a slight stretch in the base of your spine. Engaging your core muscles as this will protect your spine, pulling your pelvic floor muscles up.

2. Push your pelvis forward and bring your elbows in line with your sides.

3. Stay here for five breaths. With every out breath try deepening the back bend.

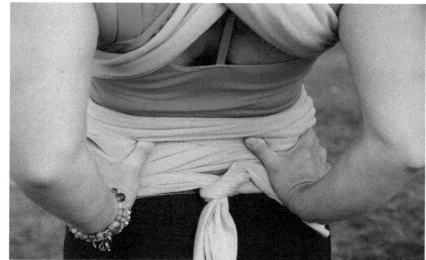

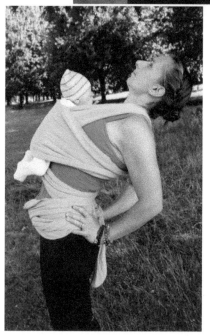

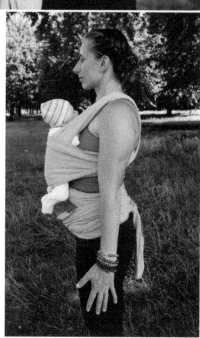

4. Inhale and bring your body back up to the centre. Releasing your arms down towards your sides.

To advance this backbend, raise both arms up together above your head, exhale and look up to your hands. Either having your arms shoulder width apart with palms facing or bring your palms together.

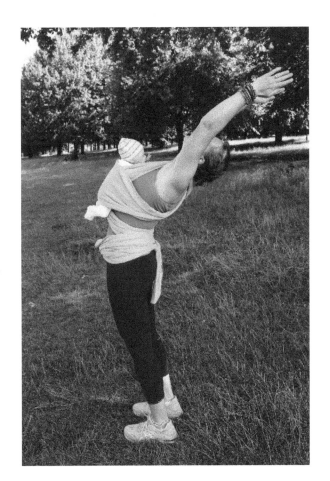

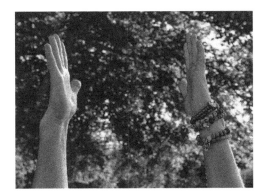

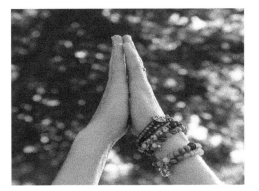

Side Bend

1. Stand in Mountain Pose and raise your arms up towards the sky. Keeping shoulders down away from your ears. Engage core muscles.

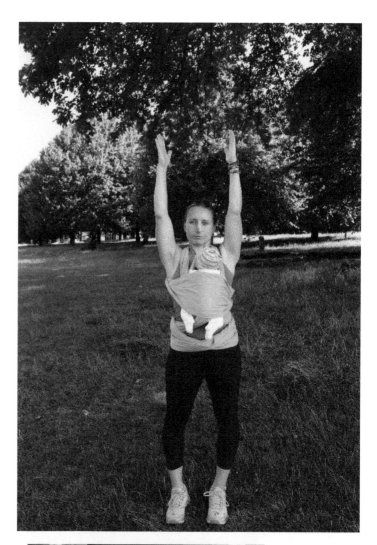

Pull up your knees activating your quadriceps (quads front thigh muscles).

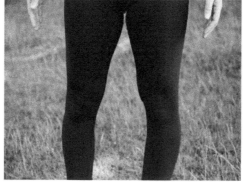

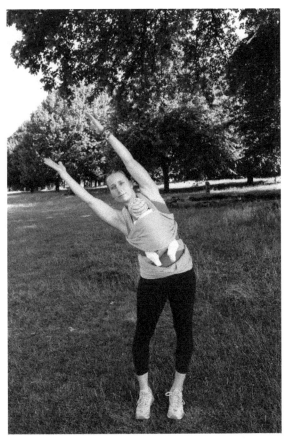

2. Exhale and fold over to one side keeping your arms raised.

3. Try to get the side of your torso to be parallel with the floor. Keeping your arms up against your ears but keep your shoulders down. Imagine you have got two panes of glass either side of you trying to keep straight. You should feel a stretch all the way down your left side of the body. Have your chest open and breathe deeply. Stay here for five breaths.

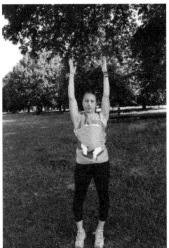

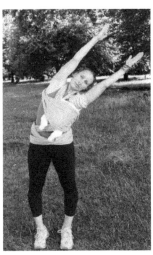

4. On your next inhale, come back up to the centre still with your arms up exhale and fold over onto the other side. Stay here for five breaths.

Page 43 Standing Side Bends

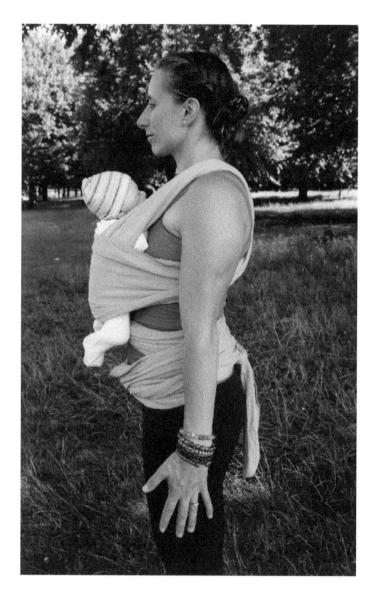

5. On your next inhale come back up to standing and exhale release your arms back down.

Tips

Be careful in these poses if you have neck injuries.

What a blessing it is to keep opening your heart when others would normally close it. – Livelifehappy.com

Head and Neck Stretch

Targets all muscles in your neck and allows a good stretch in your spine. Parents can have neck issues due to holding baby in the wrong position for your posture. This then misaligns the spine, sending everything out of sync.

Baby wearing in a wrap sat on a seat, bench or step or having baby in a buggy.

Method

1. Come into a comfortable seated position. Reach up through the crown of your head.

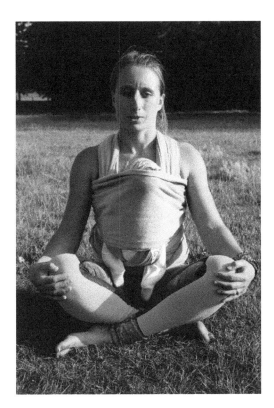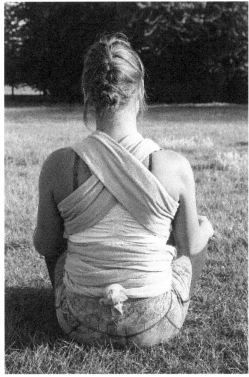

2. Keeping your back straight slowly inhale and lift your head and neck up, bringing your chin towards the sky. This creates a stretch in the front of your neck.

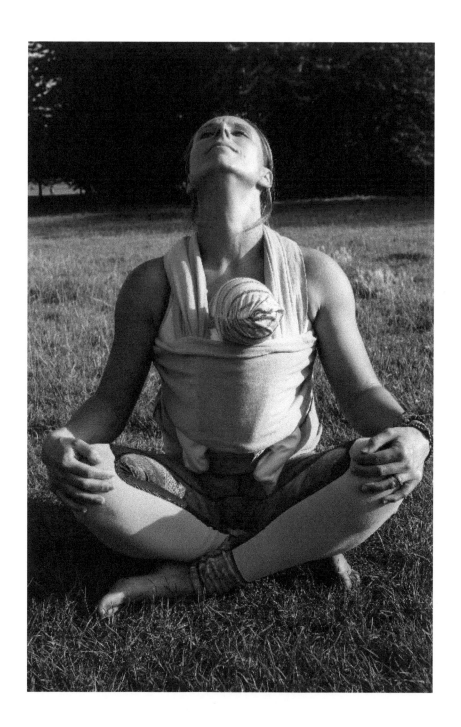

3. Exhale bringing your chin to chest. Lengthening through the back of the spine.

Repeat 5-6 times in-line with your breath. Inhale coming back to centre.

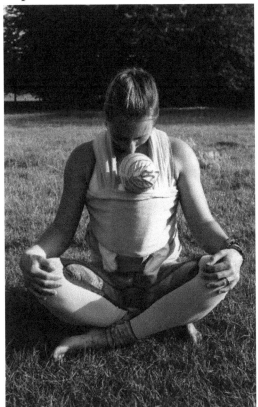 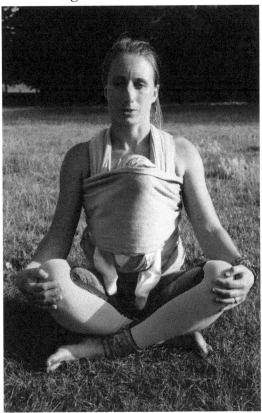

4. Exhale and turn your head over to your right shoulder, looking over your shoulder. Inhale back to centre.

5. Exhale over your left shoulder. Inhale back to centre. Repeat 5-6 times in line with your breath.

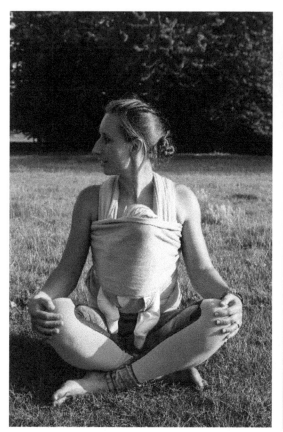 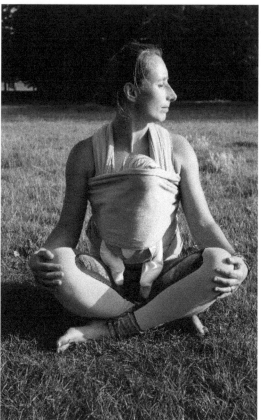

Be careful here if you have neck issues. Do not go past your comfort zone here. Just gaze to where it feels comfortable.

'Let your breath untie the knots in your body and mind' - Unknown

Cat and Cow Pose

These two poses are great for warming up your spine and allowing you to stretch out. They stretch the back, torso and neck and provide a gentle massage to the spine and internal organs.

These poses are amazing to calm your mind and to relieve stress as you are breathing with coordinating your movements. These poses are good at de stressing yourself.

Have baby on a pillow or cushion here in front of you or have him/her in the buggy. This is such a lovely pose to do to release any spinal tension especially as parents we hold our children in one arm resting on the hip.

Method

1. Come into tabletop position where your knees are stacked under your hips and your hands are stacked under your shoulders.

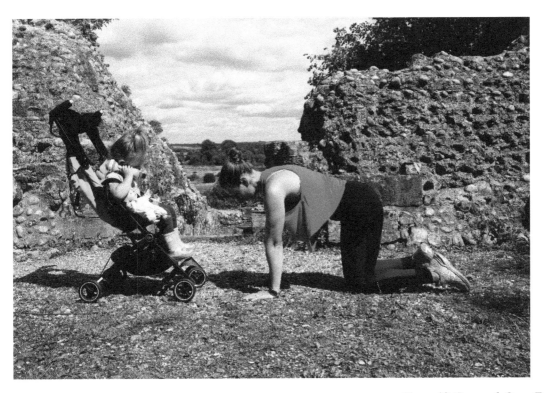

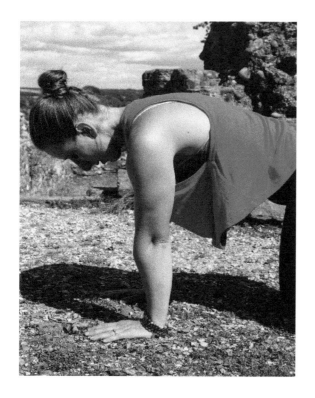 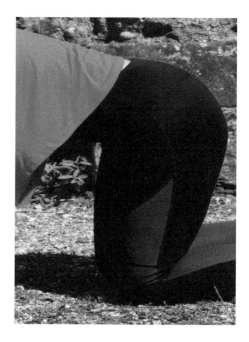

Hands are stacked under your shoulders

Knees are stacked under your hips

Let exercise be your stress reliever, not food. - Unknown

2. Have your toes pushed away from you so you are on the tops of the feet.

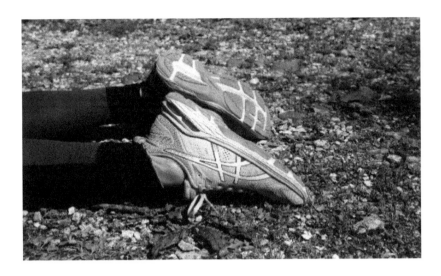

3. For some, it may be more comfortable to come onto toes.

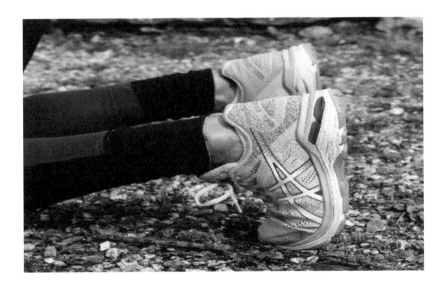

4. Inhale and go into cow pose. This is lifting the chest forward, pushing the tummy down towards the floor, lifting the tail bone up and crown of the head facing up. Relax the core muscles.

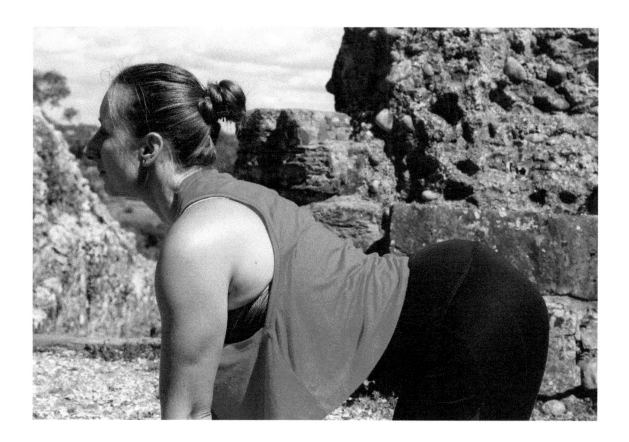

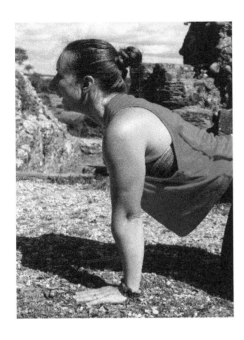

Lifting the chest forwards.

Lifting the tail bone up towards the sky.

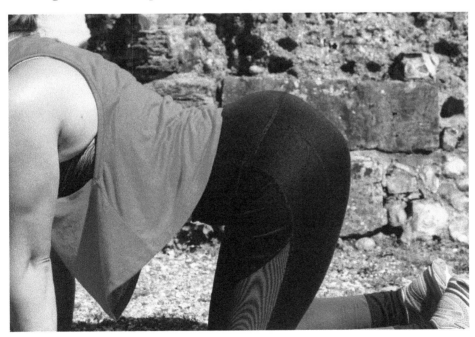

4. On an exhale come into Cat pose, tucking your head and pelvis under, rounding through your spine pushing through your hands and shoulders to round your back. Engage your core and gluteal muscles (glutes), bringing your kneecaps up into the thighs engaging the quads.

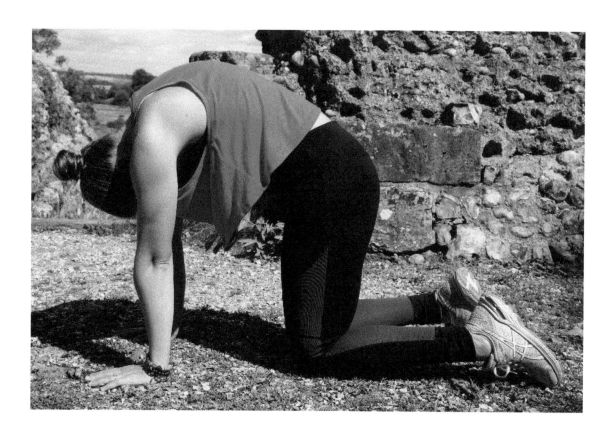

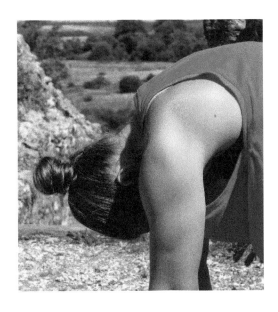

Head tucked under.

Tuck tail bone under.

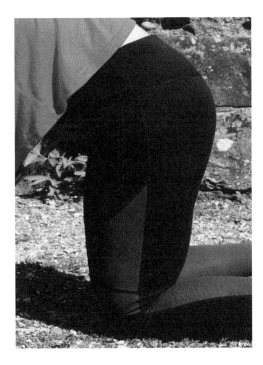

Page 55 Cat and Cow Pose

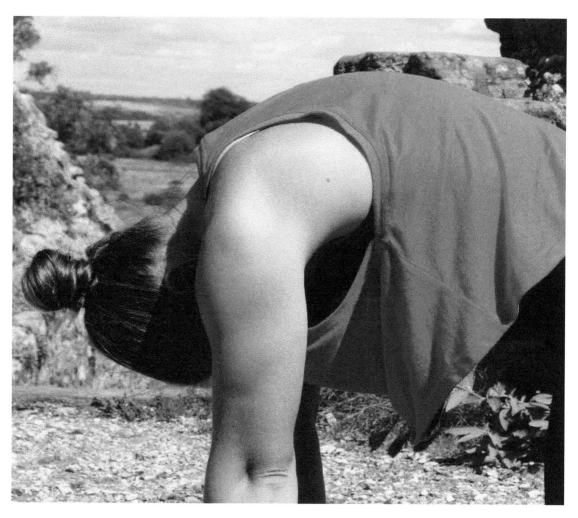

Rounding through the spine, pushing through the hands and knees.

5. Keep inhaling into cow pose and then exhaling into cat pose. Repeat these five to ten times.

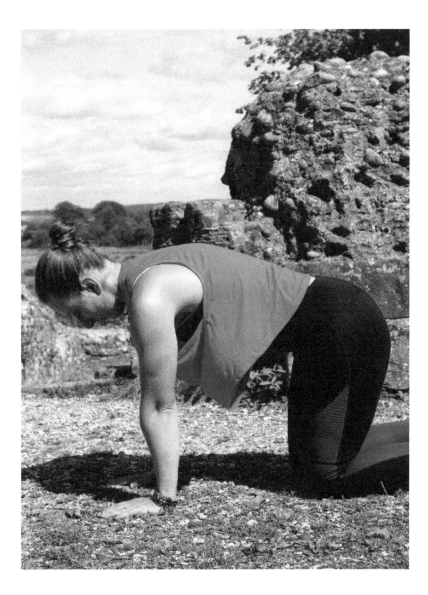

6. To come out of this pose release on an inhale from cat pose and come back into a neutral tabletop position.

Tip

If you have a neck injury, then keep your head in line with your spine and not put it up in cow pose or down in cat pose. Keep your gaze forward.

Butterfly Pose

This is a great hip opener and releases tension in your hips. A lot of people find there is so much tightness in the hips due to long periods of sitting for work. The hips will start to tighten up once the pregnancy hormones have gone from the body. This is a lovely pose to do to feel closer to your baby if putting him/her in a sling or wrap. She will feel closer to you and hear your heartbeat, relaxing her.

Method

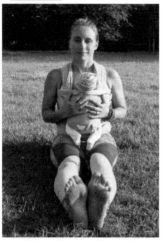

1. Come into a seated position onto the floor. Roll slightly onto the front of the sitting bones so the pubis is at the front and the tail bone is at the back. Pull out your glutes so you can feel your sit bones on the floor.

2. Bring your feet in towards you clasping your feet with your hands. Try to open out your feet like you are reading a book.

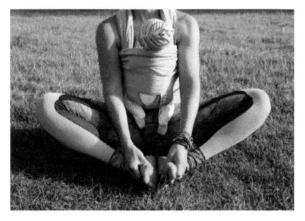

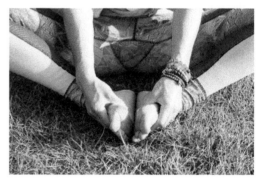

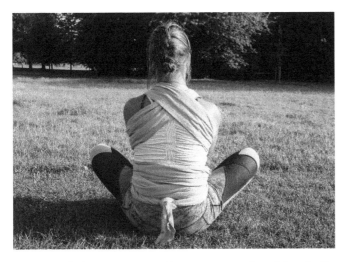

3. Lift up through the sit bones, lengthening through the spine and stretching up through the crown of your head.

4. On every exhale, move your knees out to the sides feeling the hip flexors opening, aiming to get knees parallel to the floor. Engage your core muscles and open through the chest.

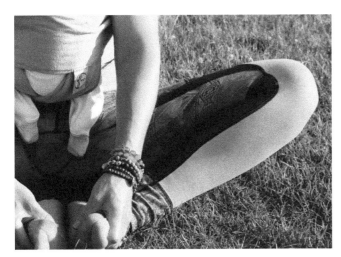

5. To advance in the pose slightly, pulse your knees outwards releasing more tension like a butterfly flapping its wings. Stay here for one to five minutes.

6. Release by bringing knees closer together and allow legs down coming back to the start position.

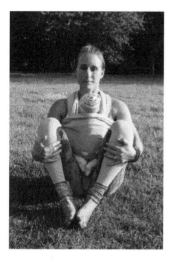 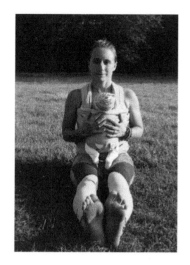

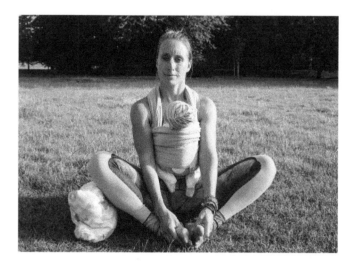

Tip

If you have got tight knees or hips here then use a block to sit on tilting the pelvis slightly forward and use blocks, cushions, or a blanket underneath each knee for support.

Be aware with any groin or knee injury.

'Just when the caterpillar thought the world was over, it became a butterfly'
— Chuang Tzu

Cow Face Arms

This is great to release tight shoulders, chest, and arms.

We as parents will always favour a stronger side when carrying baby around. This will then put more pressure on the spine and posture in general.

Shoulder openers are great to help ease the strain.

Baby can either be in a wrap or in the buggy.

Method

1. Sit kneeling with feet under your sitting bones.

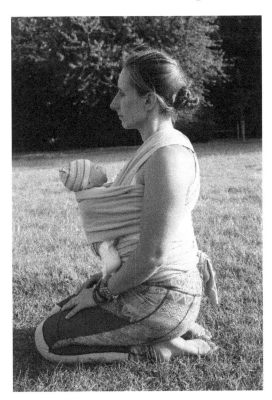

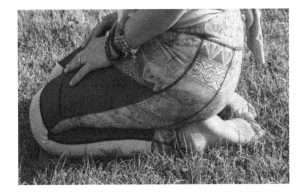

2. Keeping your back straight lifting through the crown of your head, tail bone facing towards the floor, lift one arm up to the sky and bend it with your palm facing your spine bringing your arm down your back. Keeping shoulders down and away from your ears.

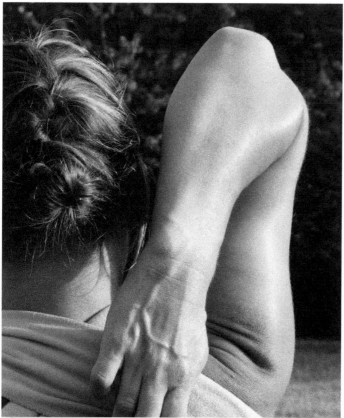

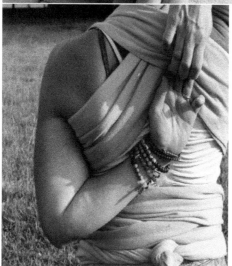

3. Bring your other arm around behind you with your palm facing outwards. Bring your hands together towards each other, clasping them if you can for a very invigorating shoulder stretch.

Page 62 Cow Face Arms

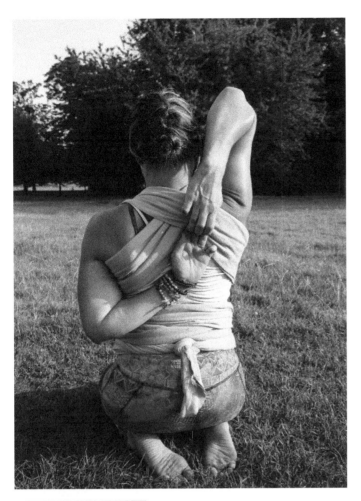

4. Try to draw the top elbow up behind the head and the bottom elbow down. This will increase the shoulders opening.

5. Release your arms and repeat on the other side.

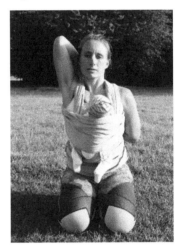

Tips

Do not do if you have serious neck or shoulder problems.

If you cannot reach your hands, then you can use a strap to get the same benefits.

One shoulder will always be tighter than the other so be careful with the tighter one.

If this is tight on your knees, then sit on a cushion with legs out in front or sit on a chair.

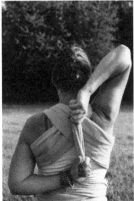

Half Forward Fold Buggy Pushouts

This exercise will help with tight hamstrings as well as helping you straighten out the spine and build up strength in the chest and shoulders.

Your baby can be in the buggy here or next to it. If using a baby wrap, then your baby's head will need to be supported as your chest will be parallel to the floor.

Method

1. Stand with your feet hip width apart about arm's length away from the buggy.

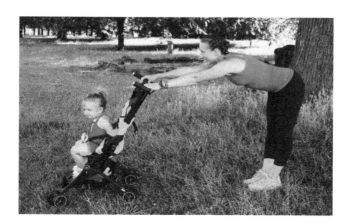 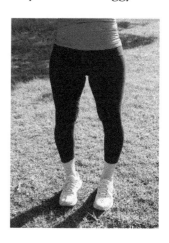

2. Bring your palms together in prayer position.

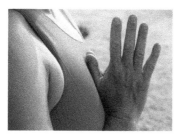

Engage your gluteal muscles (glutes), pull knees up into thighs engaging your quads. Engage the core and spread out your toes evenly.

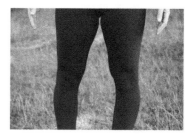

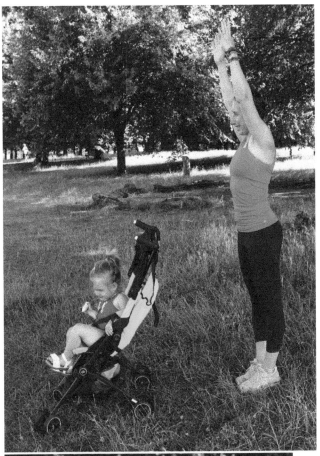

4. As you inhale, raise your arms overhead, keeping your palms facing towards each other. Either have your hands shoulder width apart or together sliding the shoulders down away from your ears.

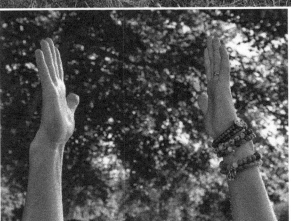

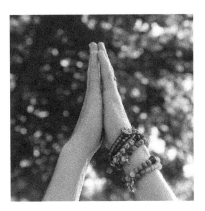

5. Exhale diving forward keeping the back flat bringing your fingertips to the floor. If your hands do not touch your feet, then just go as far as is comfortable bringing your hands towards the shins.

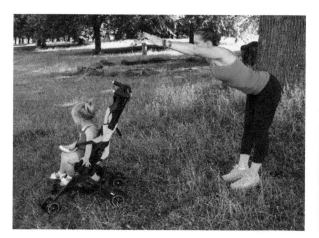
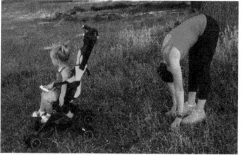

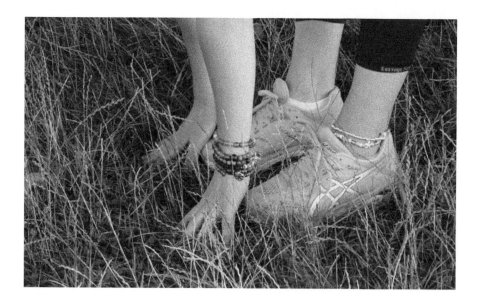

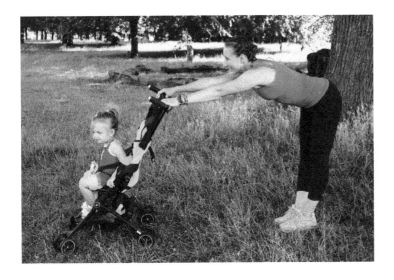

6. Inhale look up and lengthen having a straight back. Sending your hips backwards, keeping the legs engaged.

7. Bring your arms parallel to the buggy holding onto the handle.

8. Bring the buggy towards your chest bending at the elbows.

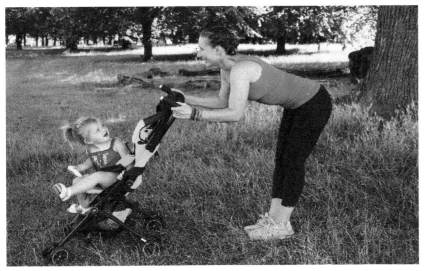

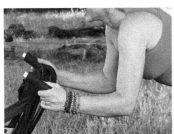

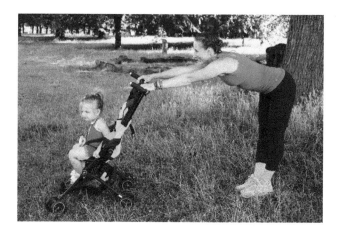

9. Then push back out to have straight arms.

10. Repeat these ten to fifteen times.

11. Come out releasing hands and pushing back up to standing.

Tip

To advance this exercise come onto tip toes and push out with your arms. This will build up strength in your calves.

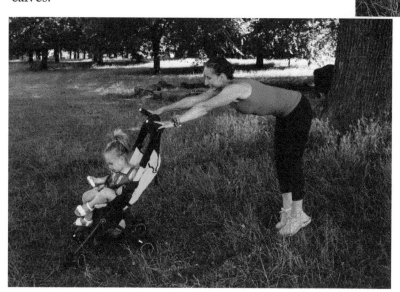

You don't need:

A fancy gym, Nikes, Or new sweatpants to exercise.

You just need yourself, your baby and some motivation -
Unknown

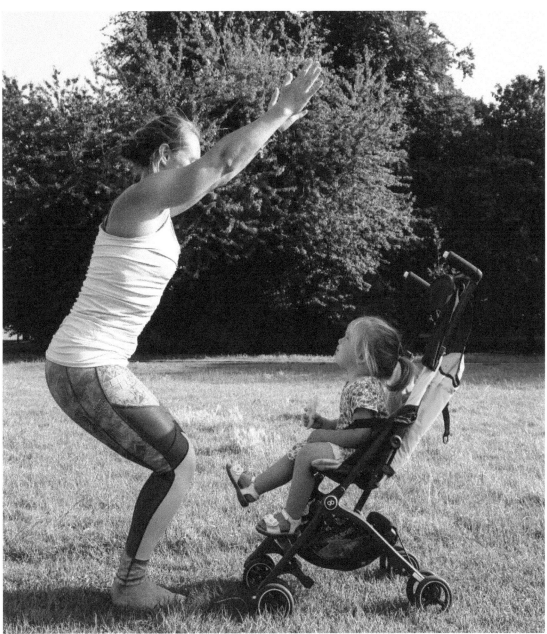

Figure 2 - Chair Pose with Baby in Buggy.

Chapter Four

Sun Salutation A

Sun Salutation B

Sun Salutation A

Sun Salutations are a series of poses put together in a sequence where you inhale for one pose and exhale into the next pose. This is a good sequence of poses to warm up and improves overall health and wellbeing. Depending on how fast or slow you do them, will depend on how you feel at the end of it. If you do this sequence fast, you will feel energised and if you do this sequence slow you will feel calm and in a meditative state ready to face anything life throws at you (especially with children).

<u>**Method**</u>   Have your baby in the buggy or next to you in the sequence.

1. Stand in mountain Pose (See page 35 for more information). Bring your palms together in prayer position.

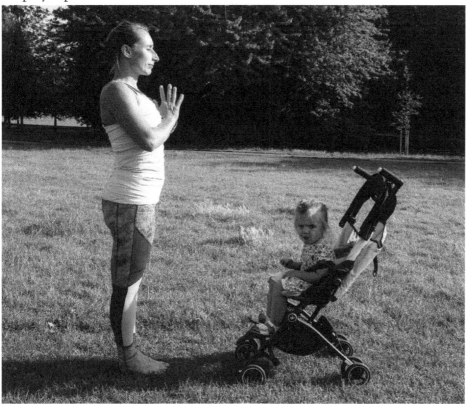

2. Engage your gluteal muscles (glutes), pull knees up into thighs engaging your quads. Engage the core and spread out your toes evenly.

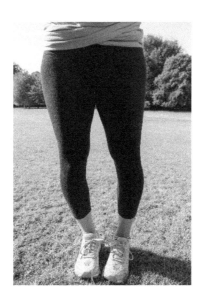

3. Inhale, raising your arms overhead, keeping your palms facing towards each other. Either have your hands shoulder width apart or together sliding the shoulders down away from your ears.

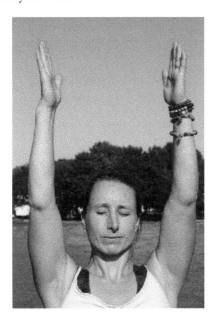

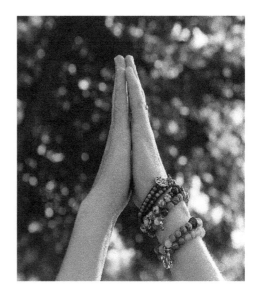

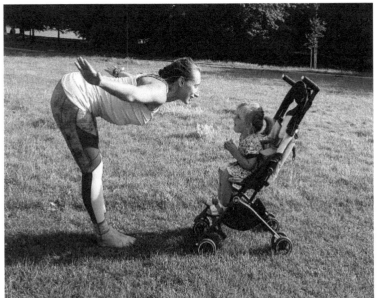

4. Exhale diving forward keeping the back flat bringing your fingertips to the floor. If your hands do not touch your feet, then just go as far as is comfortable bringing your hands towards the shins.

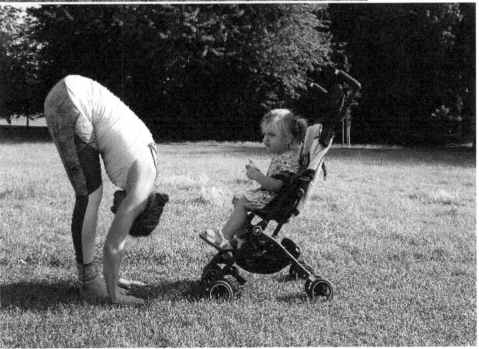

Hands to floor or onto shins.

5. Inhale look up having a straight back. Sending your hips backwards, keeping the legs engaged.

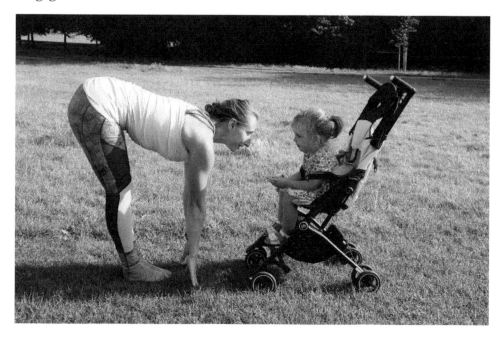

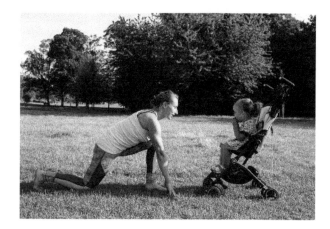

6. Exhaling, step or jump both legs back so you are in a high plank position. Come down onto your knees first if that feels better. Keep your spine and legs in a straight line and support your weight on hands and feet.

Onto knees or go to plank position pushing the ground away from you.

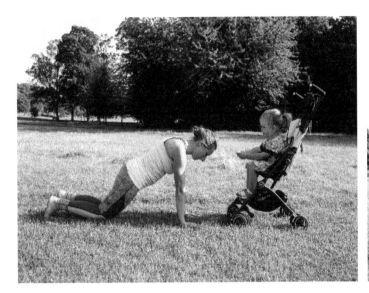

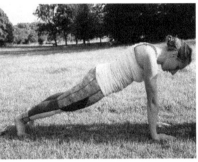

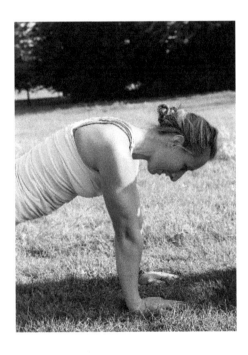

Have your hands stacked under your shoulders fingers spread wide.

7. Lower yourself down into Low plank or chaturanga keeping the elbows in towards the chest. Coming onto your knees first to avoid the strain in your lower back, then lower the chest and chin towards the floor.

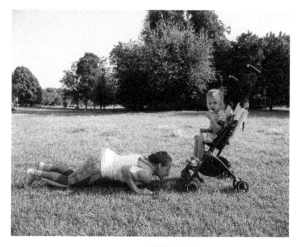

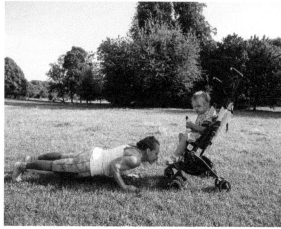

8. Inhale and push yourself forwards into Upward facing Dog. Push your pelvis down towards the floor, pushing your chest forwards and gazing forwards. Bring the tops of your feet onto the floor and press through your hands. This will open your chest.

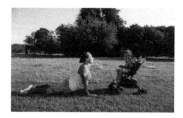

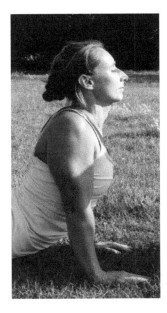
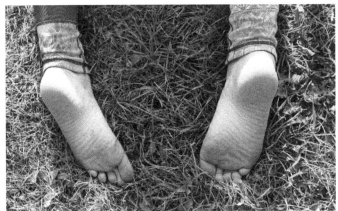

Chest lifted and tops of the feet onto the floor.

9. Exhale, curl your toes back under, press down into your heels, and lift your hips so you are in Downward facing Dog. Stay here for five breaths. (See page 159 For information on how to do Downward facing dog).

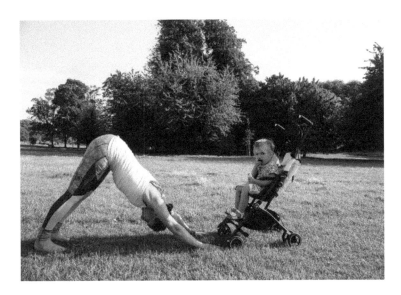

10. Come up onto your toes, lift your hips into the air, bend your knees and gaze through to your hands.

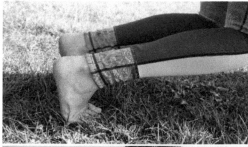

Onto toes.

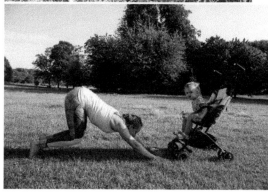

11. On your next exhale step forward to bring your feet to your hands. You will end up in forward fold.

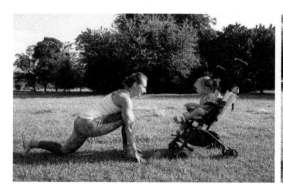 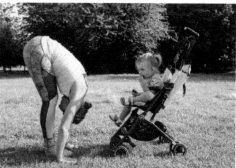

12. Inhale and come into halfway lift gazing forward keeping your back flat.

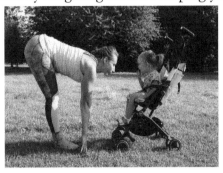

Exhale forward fold again then coming back up arms out to the side's back to mountain pose.

Repeat as many times as you like.

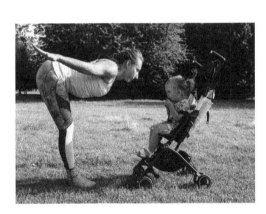
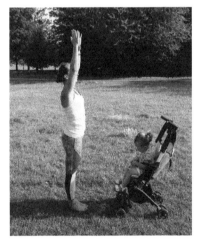

Tip

Be aware of any back, wrist or knee problems here and high blood pressure.

If any wrist issues, then when in Downward facing dog come into your forearms to release the pressure in your wrists.

Even if you can't physically see the results in front of you right now, every single effort you do is changing your body from the inside. Never get discouraged! - Unknown

Sun Salutation B

This is a good sequence of poses to warm you up and improves overall health and wellbeing. Depending on how fast or slow you do them, will depend on how you feel at the end of it. If you do this sequence fast, you will feel energised and if you do this sequence slow you will feel calm and in a meditative state ready to face anything life throws at you (especially with children).

Method
1. Stand in Chair Pose (see page 112 for instructions on how to do this).

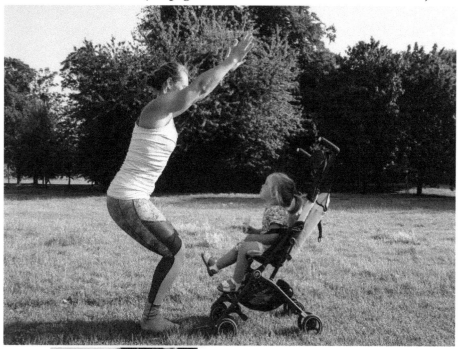

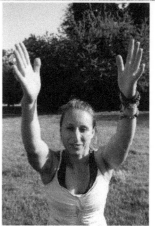

2. As you inhale, raise your arms overhead, keeping your palms facing towards each other. Either have your hands shoulder width apart or together sliding the shoulders down away from your ears. Trying to create a lightning bolt shape.

3. Exhale diving forward keeping the back flat bringing your fingertips to the floor. If your hands do not touch your feet, bring your hands towards the shins. Also straightening out the legs.

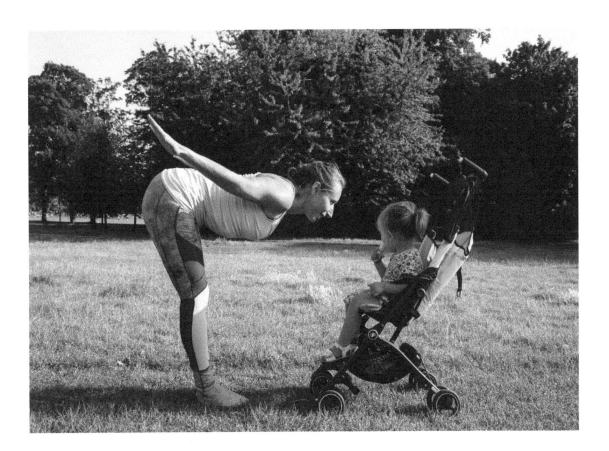

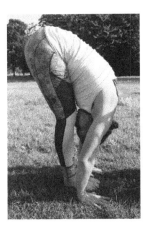

Bringing the head down towards your knees.

4. Inhale look up and lengthen having a straight back. Sending your hips backwards, keeping the muscles in the legs engaged.

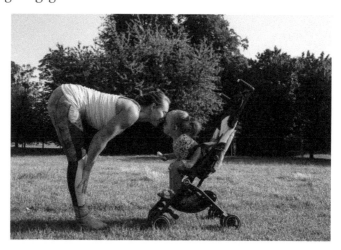

5. Exhaling, step or jump both legs back so you are in a high plank position. Come down onto your knees first if that feels better and is safer for diastasis recti. Keep your spine and legs in a straight line and support your weight on hands and feet. Have your hands stacked under your shoulders, fingers spread wide.

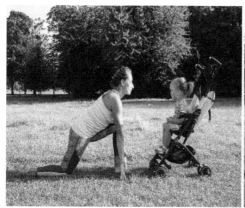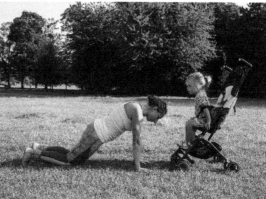

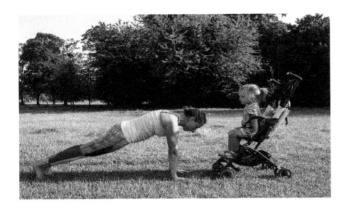 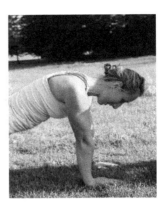

6. Lower yourself down into Low plank or chaturanga keeping the elbows in towards the chest. Coming onto your knees first to avoid the strain in your lower back, then lower the chest and chin towards the floor.

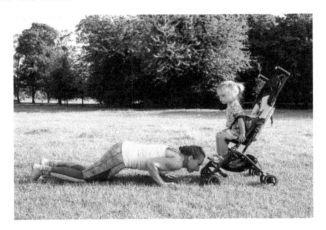

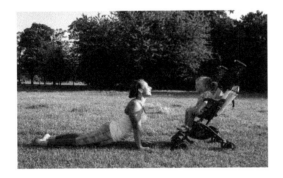

7. Inhale and push yourself forwards into Upward facing Dog. Push your pelvis down towards the floor, pushing your chest forwards and gazing forwards. Bring the tops of your feet onto the floor and press through your hands. This will open your chest.

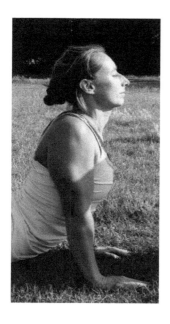

Chest lifted and tops of the feet onto the floor.

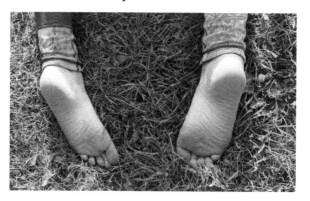

8. Exhale, curl your toes back under, bend through your knees, press down into your heels, and lift your hips so you are in Downward facing Dog. (See page 159 For information on how to do Downward facing dog).

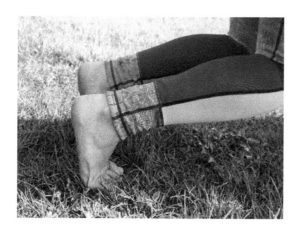

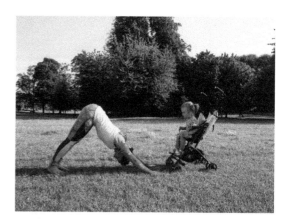

9. On an inhale engage your core and bring the right foot through to your hands, helping it through if you need to. Press into the outside of the back foot and bring your torso and arms up, bending the front knee to come into Warrior One. Check that your knee is not folding in on itself and have your knee stacked over the ankle. Engage your glutes here, pulling pelvic floor muscles up.

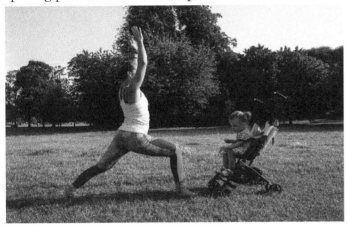

Have knee over ankle and check you can see your big toe while looking down the inside of your front knee.

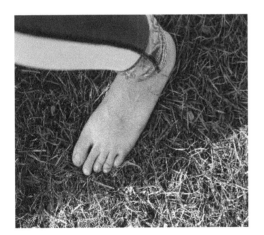 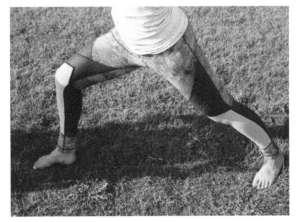

10. On your exhale come back to high plank and repeat stages five to nine again but swapping to the left leg.

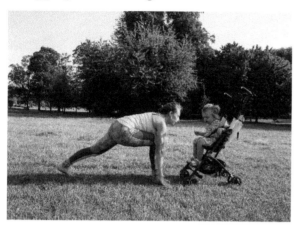 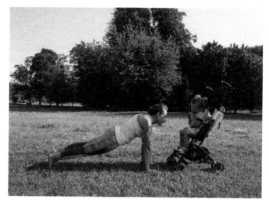

11. Repeat stages five to eight once more ending in downward facing dog.

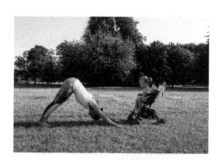

12. Come up onto your toes, lift your hips into the air, bend your knees and gaze through to your hands. On your next exhale step forward to bring your feet through to your hands. Bring feet together, having knees, ankles and thighs touching. You will end up in forward fold.

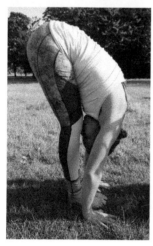

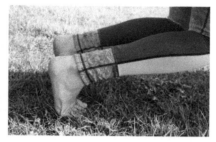

13. Inhale and come into halfway lift gazing forward keeping your back flat.

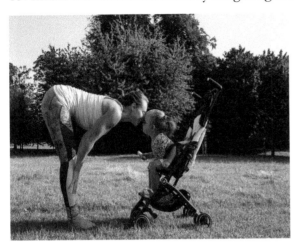 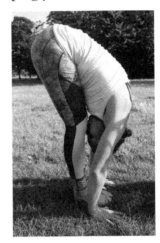

14. Exhale forward fold again.

15. On an inhale coming back up a with bent knees to Chair pose, bringing the arms up over your head to create a lightning bolt pose. Exhale and release back to standing.

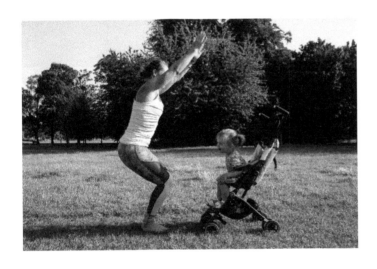

16. Repeat as many times as you like.

Tip

Be aware of any back, wrist or knee problems here and high blood pressure.

If you have any wrist issues, then when in Downward facing dog come onto your forearms to release the pressure in your wrists.

'You will never always be motivated, so you must learn to be disciplined'
- Unknowm

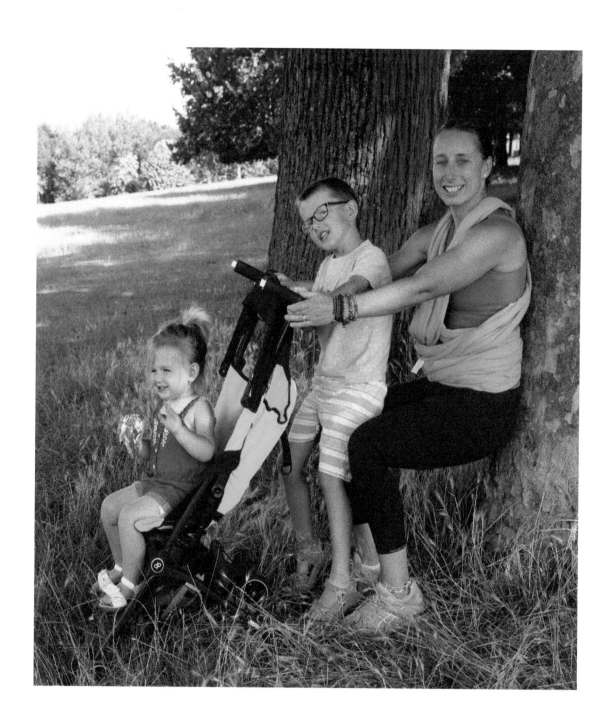

Chapter Five

Baby Wearing either in a wrap or sling (if this includes both e.g. using a buggy as well, then this is stated)

Step up's and Step up Side Kicks

Tree Pose

Bridge Pose and Bridge Touches with a buggy

Boat V Sit

Camel Pose

Tricep Dips

Chair Pose

Hand to Knee Pose

Low Lunge

High Lunge and Walking Lunges

Wall Sit

Chest Press

Step ups and Step Up Side Kick

These are a great way to help strengthen your glutes (buttocks) and work your hamstrings (muscles at the back of your thighs) quadriceps (muscles at the front of your thighs) and core. They also can help strengthen your lower and middle spine.

We must be mindful with regards to our spine and lift correctly bending our knees and keeping our spine straight. These Step ups will help in increase overall strength and build a stronger foundation with lifting child in mind. With or without your baby in a wrap.

Method Step Up

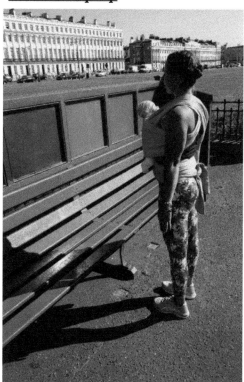

1. Using a solid base for example a step, chair or park bench stand about a foot away from it. Feet hip width apart.

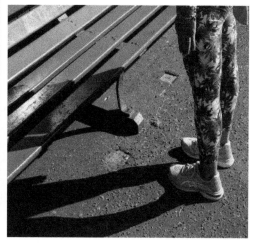

2. Engage your standing leg muscles and core and begin to move the other leg, stepping up onto the step or box.

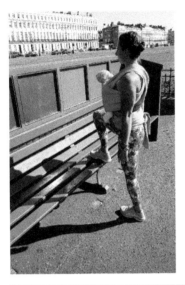

3. Drive through the heel and push the other leg up onto the step, keeping your hip and knees stable and correctly aligned.

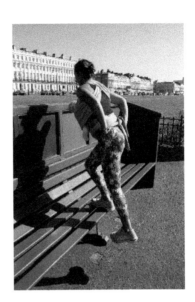

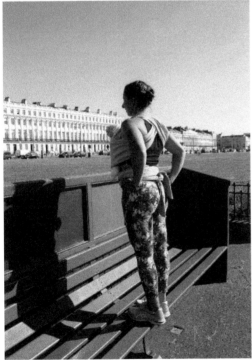

4. Stand on the step or box with both feet. Keeping core and legs engaged.

5. Start to lower the other leg back down to the ground, keeping core engaged. Do not let it just fall. Slowly lower back down to the ground.

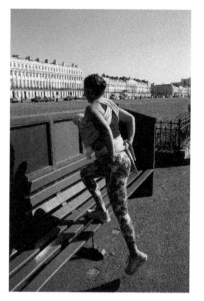 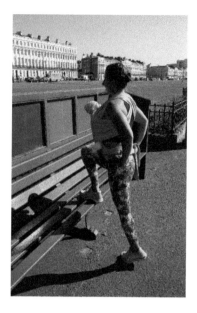

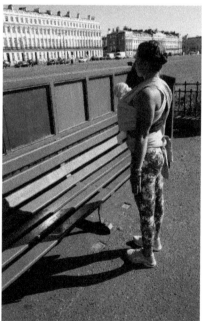

6. Repeat with the other leg lowering back down and repeat aiming for ten to fifteen reps.

Method Step Up Side Kick

1. Follow steps one and two

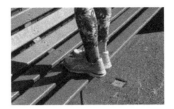

2. With both feet on the step slightly bend one leg and shift your weight to that standing leg.

3. Slowly lift the other leg off the step and engaging leg muscles propel that leg out to the side.

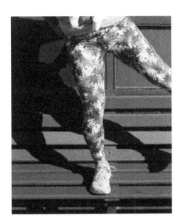 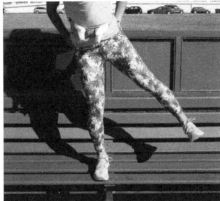

4. Bringing it back to the start and repeat on the other side.

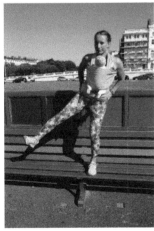

Tip
Be careful of knee joints here. Make sure your knee is stacking over your ankle and no further forward. If it is bringing your foot back slightly to align your knee.

Advance this exercise
Add in some weights for example light dumbbells or baked bean can if doing this at home.

'A little progress each day adds up to big results' - Diana Martin

Tree pose Baby Wearing or holding onto

Tree pose is an all-round fantastic posture. It stretches out your entire body. It strengthens thighs, calves, ankles, and spine. It stretches the groin, inner thighs and pelvis, chest, and shoulders. All of which are needed when carrying baby around or in life in general.

It improves sense of balance, relieves sciatica, and reduces flat feet. It also builds concentration and balance.

Method   1. Start in mountain pose, (Go to page 35 to find method of Mountain pose) find a fixed gaze point just in front of you.

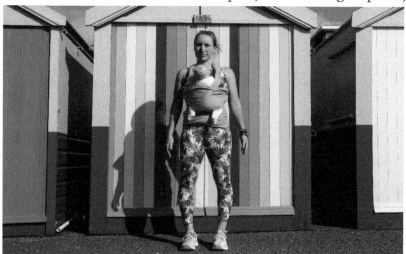

2. Engage your core muscles (go to page 94 for information about the core), tucking pelvis slightly under.

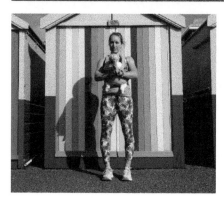

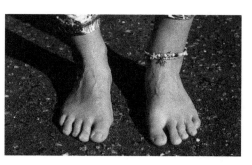

3. Spread your standing toes wide, feeling all four corners of the ground around your foot. Bring your kneecap slightly up on your standing leg so you are engaging your quads (Quadriceps muscles are the front of your thighs).

4. Find your gaze point just in front of you or at your eye line in front. As you shift your weight through to the standing foot, slightly start to lift off the other foot, placing it on your inner calf or thigh.

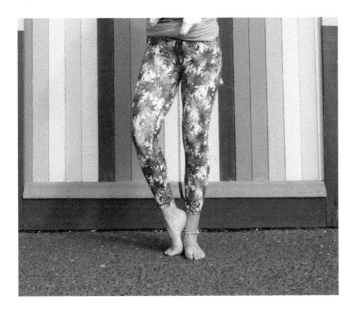

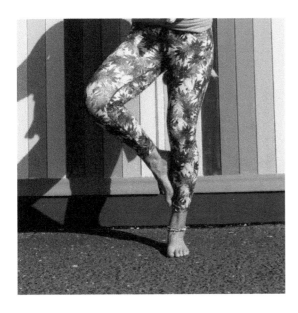

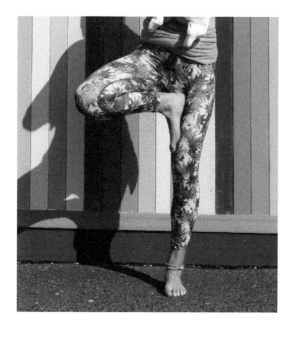

5. On your bent knee, have your toes pointing towards the floor. Press your heel into the inner side of the thigh or calf.

6. Rest your hands on your pelvis to start with, then bring your hands into prayer position in front of your chest or bring them above your head keeping shoulders away from ears.

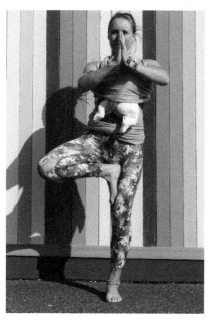

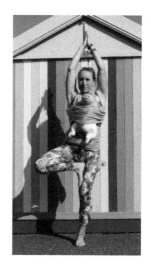

7. Stay here for up to one minute. Come back to the centre and repeat on the other side.

Tip

Easier version holding onto buggy, wall, or anything stable.

You should not try Tree pose if you have got high or low blood pressure, suffer from insomnia, or have migraines. Make sure your baby is secure in the wrap or carrier before continuing in this pose.

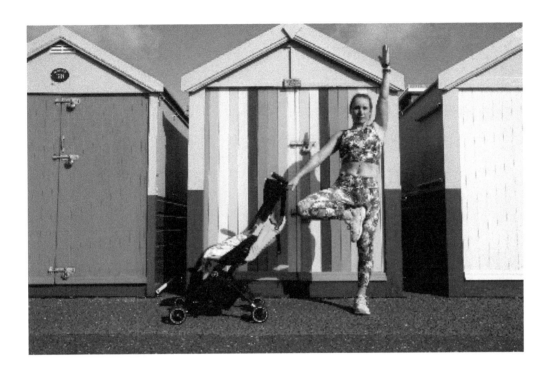

Advice from a Tree, Stall tall and proud, Sink your roots into the earth

Be content with your natural beauty, Go out on a limb,

Drink plenty of water, Remember your roots

Enjoy the view! (Ilan Shamin)

Bridge and Bridge Touches - Baby Wearing or with a Buggy

This is good for strengthening the spine, hands and wrists. It opens the chest and is a great weight loss/ fat burner from the stomach as you stretch further into the pose. It also fires up your gluteal muscles (glutes). This can also be a very energising pose to be in and parents may like this to relax in.

You can have you baby in a wrap or in the buggy for this exercise.

Method

1. Lie on your back with your knees bent hip width apart and feet flat on the floor, bringing the feet as close to your pelvis as you want to go.

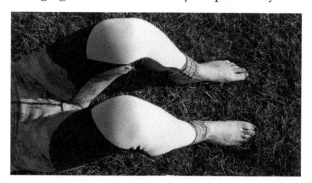

2. Have your palms facing towards the floor.

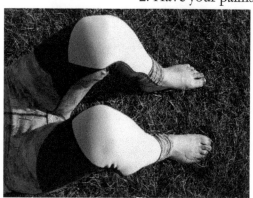 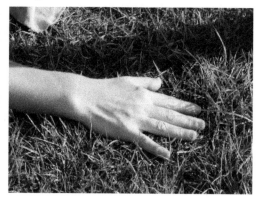

3. On your next inhale, push up through your forearms and hands engaging your glutes, core and leg muscles. Peeling your pelvis off the floor vertebrae by vertebrae and lifting through your pelvis.

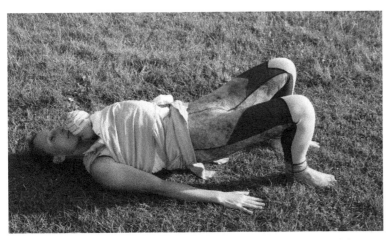

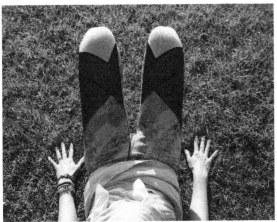
Knees falling out to the sides - Wrong

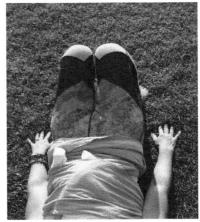
Knees falling inwards - Wrong

4. Keep pushing into your forearms and hands. Make sure that your knees are not falling in or out to the sides. Keep them strong and stacked over the ankles.

5. Engage your glutes and keep pushing up to get your pelvis as far away from the floor as possible. Wriggle your shoulders slightly under your back. Lift the chin slightly away from your chest. Stay here for five breaths.

6. If you wish you can take it a bit further and interlace your fingers underneath your spine, wriggling your shoulders further under and lifting through the spine further. This will give you a stronger stretch in your glutes.

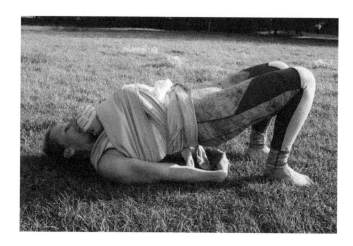

7. If you want to advance even further, release one leg off from the floor and bring it up into the air pointing your foot to the sky or pushing the heel away engaging your calf muscles.

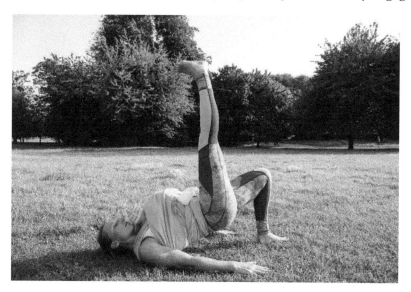

8. To come out of the pose on an exhale, slowly release your spine and pelvis back down into the floor vertebrae by vertebrae.

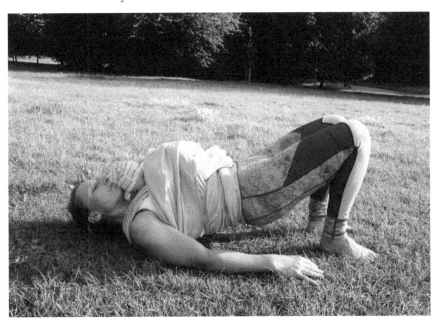

9. Once on the floor, slowly hug your knees into your chest to release your back and rock from side to side, keeping the tail bone down. towards the floor.

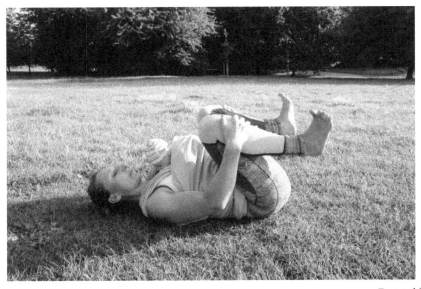

Bridge Touches - With a Buggy

Follow the same as above but instead of having feet flat on the floor, have one foot placed onto the foot plate of the buggy. Keeping core and legs engaged, touch the buggy with that foot, then lower that foot back down and raise the other leg to come onto the foot plate. Keeping the bridge always formed.

To advance this further, slowly push the buggy away drawing it back and forth with each leg for five to ten times. Slowly release to come out.

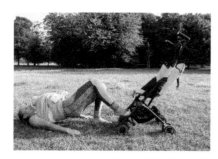 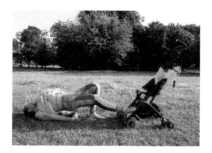

If you advance this further, then this will really fire up your glutes making them burn more fat around that area.

For a restorative bridge, place a block or cushion under the spine by your pelvis just above the knicker line. Have your hands down by your pelvis and rest here for however long you need to. This will direct the blood flow towards the heart and head where it is needed the most. To come out, release the block and gently hug knees into chest releasing the lower spine. Keep the tail bone and pubis down towards the floor.

A fun add on to this pose is to come into a bridge following the instructions above, holding your baby in up in front of you or so they are resting on your tummy if they are not in the buggy. Keep baby here and lower down. Raise back up again repeating five to ten times keeping the correct form.

Tip

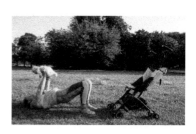

Be careful in this pose if you have neck problems.

Imagine a piece of string attached to your pelvis lifting you up higher.

It does not matter how slowly you go as long as you do not stop. - Confucius

Page 102 Bridge Pose

Boat V-Sit - Either Baby Wearing or in a Buggy

This is a great exercise to tone and strengthen your abdominal muscles. It can also improve your overall balance and concentration. It strengthens your spine and hip flexors and lengthens the hamstrings.

You can have your baby in a wrap attached to your chest, hold your baby in front of you or have him/her in a buggy.

Method

1. Come into a seated position, legs out in front of you. Pull your buttocks away from you so you are sitting on your sitting bones. Have your hands down by your sides.

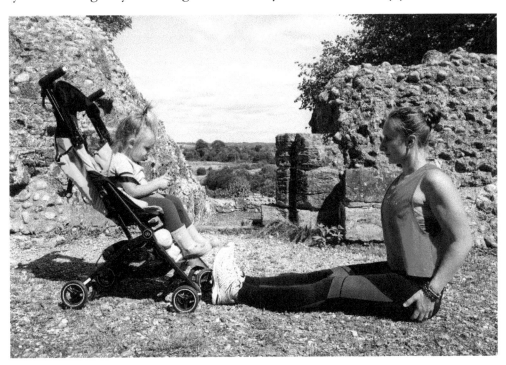

2. Engage your core muscles pulling pelvic floor muscles up into the abdomen. Keep your chest lifted drawing the shoulder blades backwards and slide them down your back. Roll onto the back of your sit bones.

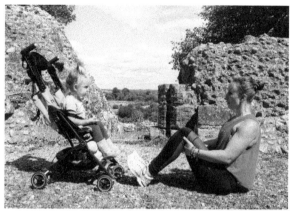

3. Keeping core engaged, bend your knees, and hold onto the back of them. Slowly start to lift your feet off from the floor. Try not to collapse in your lower back, keeping the chest pushed forwards.

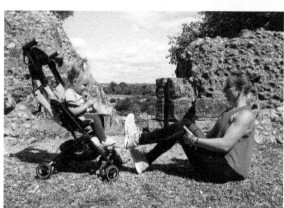

4. Squeeze your knees together, engaging all your leg muscles. Breath and stay here for ten to fifteen breaths.

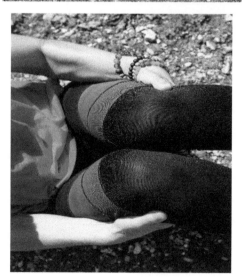

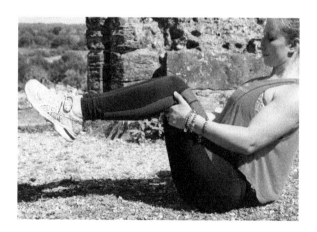

Page 104 Boat Pose V Sit

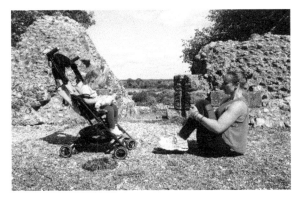

5. Slowly release and come back to the start.

Tip

Be kind to your pelvic floor in this exercise. Try gently to engage them building strength up as your baby gets older.

Be careful here if you have a healing Diastasis Recti. This pose is not advisable if you still have quite a large gap.

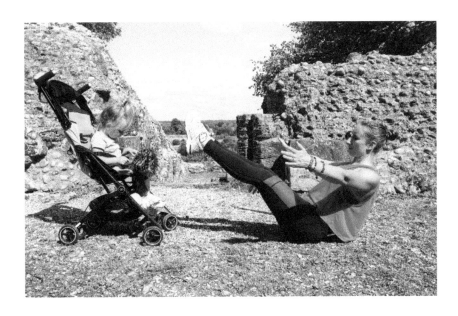

To advance this exercise from the normal position, straighten your legs out and bring your hands away from your knees with palms facing towards your legs, engaging arm muscles. Keep your shoulders down away from yours ears.

Boat V Sit - Using a Buggy

Assume position above but place feet on the buggy foot plate. Drawing legs in and out always engaging your core.

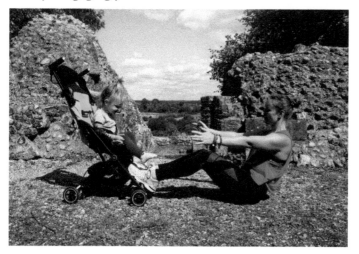

Slowly release and come back to the start.

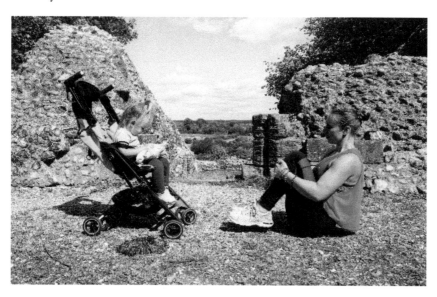

If the ocean can calm itself, so can you. We are both salt water mixed with air. – Nayyirah Waheed

Camel pose

This pose is great to stretch out the entire front of the body including ankles, thighs and groin, abdomen, chest, and throat.

It stretches the deep hip flexors, strengthening the back muscles and improves posture, it also stimulates the organs of the abdomen and neck, and can help with anxiety and mild backache.

Baby can be in a baby wrap or in the buggy next to you.

Method

1.Come up onto your knees, keeping them hip width apart, pressing your shins and tops of feet firmly into the floor, stacking your pelvis over your knees. Engage your quadriceps (quads-front thigh muscles) by bringing kneecaps up into thighs. Draw your thighs in slightly and have your pelvis slightly tilted up so tail bone is down.

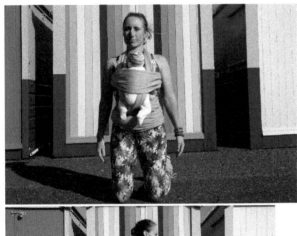

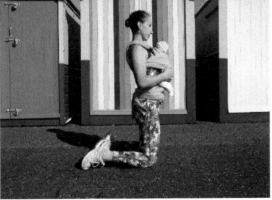

2. Bring your hands behind and place them on your hips with your palms facing inwards, fingers pointing around your waist, thumbs pointing towards your spine.

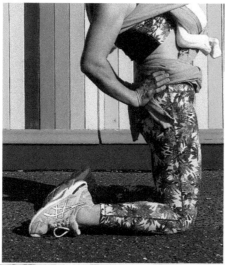

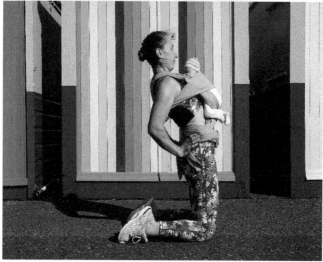

3. Exhale and arch your spine backwards, pressing your hands in towards your spine. Let your head hang back a little. Be careful here if you have neck issues. Press your thighs forwards and arch in the lower back.

4. Stay here for five breaths.

5. Come out on your next exhale and fold forward slightly to release any tension in your lower back.

Advanced pose

Follow the method above but release your hands towards your ankles, pushing your pelvis forwards and bringing the shoulders towards each other. Aim to touch or have fingers on the tops of heels, pushing against feet.

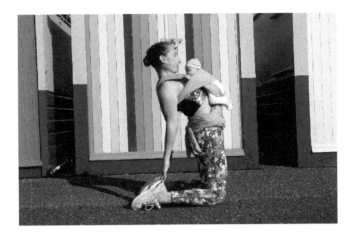

Tips

Do not do this pose if you have lower back issues. Do not push your head backwards if you have neck problems. Keep your head lifted or use a wall and rest your head against the wall or buggy.

Try not to let your lower ribs face the sky as this puts pressure on your lower spine. A good tip here is to try this against a wall, trying to keep your thighs pressed against it and lean back, this way you are getting the full benefits without hurting the lower spine.

Be careful in the pose if you have high or low blood pressure which has not been treated.

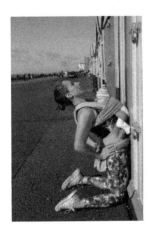

'The yoga pose that you avoid the most, you need the most.'- Unknown

Page 109 Camel Pose

Tricep Dips

Tricep Dips are great for building up upper body strength especially triceps (muscles at the back of your upper arm) and shoulders. You can do them anywhere. All you need is a chair, bench, or step. When carrying our children around we need strong arms and core to protect our lower spine.

Method

1. Position yourself on the bench with your hands behind your back in line with your hips with your fingers facing forwards and slightly off the chair or bench. Keeping your feet and knees hip distance apart.

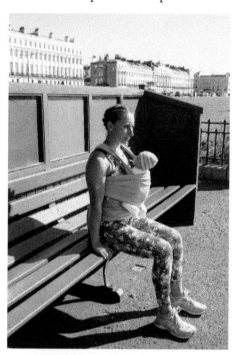

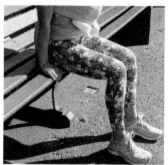

2. Walk your feet about a foot away from where you were originally positioned and start bending your elbows, keeping elbows in line with your chest. Keep your upper arms and core engaged.

3. On an exhale, drive through your hands and heels, start to lower your body down to a 90-degree angle, keeping your back straight and aiming your tail bone (coccyx) towards the floor. Do not touch the floor. Sending the elbows backwards but still in line with chest. Keep knees positioned over ankles so as not to put too much pressure on knees.

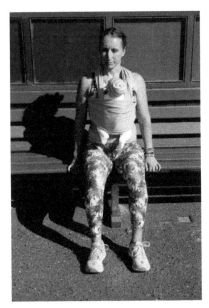
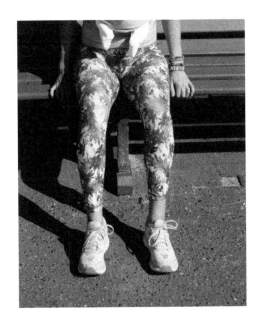
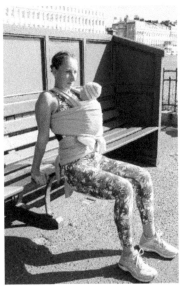
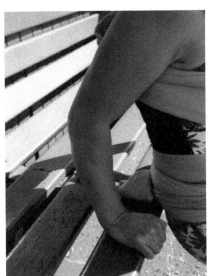

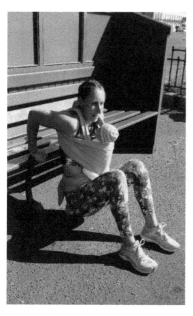

4. On an out breath, slowly come back up, keeping your shoulders wrapped around your back and keeping the chest lifted, straightening elbows to come into the start position.

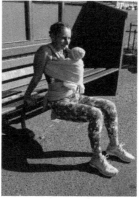

5. Repeat five to ten times.

For a slightly harder version keep legs straight and lower down the same way.

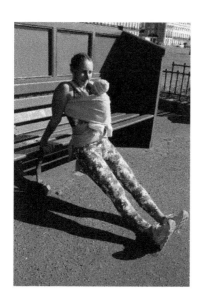

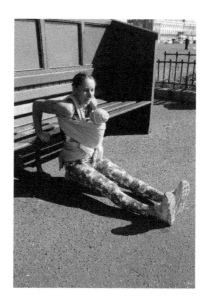

Tip

Be aware of any pre-existing shoulder injuries. This exercise helps to use the muscles around the back and shoulders and does not put pressure on the joints.

'Exercise not only changes your body. It changes your mind, your attitude and your mood.' - Unknown

Chair Pose - Wearing Baby or in a Buggy

This pose is amazing at strengthening your legs and arms. It also allows your chest to be open, helping you to breathe correctly.

You can have your baby here in a wrap on your chest or in the buggy. If baby is in the buggy, try the advanced version for a leg workout.

Method

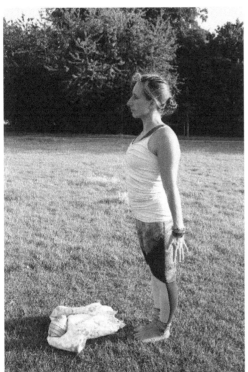

1. Stand up straight with your legs together. Keep your feet, ankles, and knees in a line. Have arms by your sides. Engage all your leg muscles.

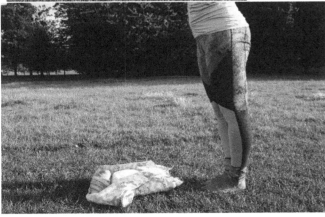

2. On an inhale, bend your knees and swing your arms up over your head. Bring your palms to face each other, shoulder width apart or bring palms together. Push your shoulders down away from your ears.

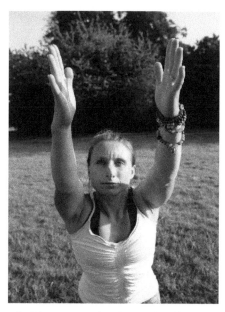 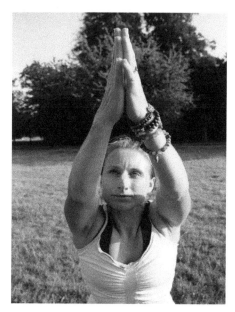

3. Keep your heels on the floor, slightly rolling into the back of them. Aim to have your tail bone tucked under, keeping your lower back long. Aim to get your thighs parallel towards the floor. Engage your core. Pull your pelvic floor muscles up. Check you can see your toes, making sure your knees are not protruding over them.

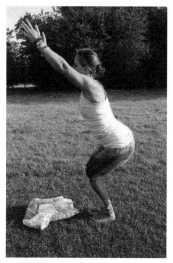 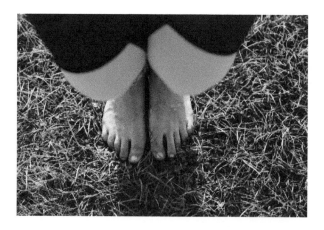

4. Breathe through the pose, take a big inhale and exhale. On every exhale try and sink a bit lower to the floor, bending your knees slightly again. Slightly arch your back.

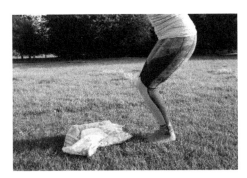

This pose is very strong on your thighs and arms. Breathe and it becomes easier.

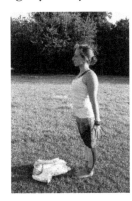

5. To come out of this pose straighten your legs on an inhale and release your arms back down to your sides.

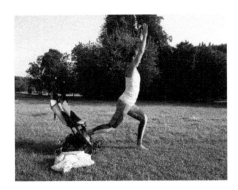

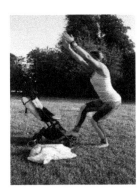

Another option is to use the footplate of the buggy for a quad workout.

To advance this pose using the buggy, place one foot onto the foot pad of the buggy behind you. Push it away, bending the other leg further towards the floor keeping the correct alignment. Bring the leg back up to the front and repeat five times on each leg. This will really activate your glutes (buttocks) and quadriceps (front of thigh). Come back up to the start position and swap legs. Notice the burn.

Tips

Do not do this pose if you have low blood pressure.

Using a wall or bench, stand close to the wall with your back facing towards it. Lower down into Chair Pose with your tail bone just touching the wall. Use the wall to rest here if need be and to get the correct alignment.

'It takes a big heart to shape little minds.' -
Unknown

Hand to Knee Pose

This pose is great to improve your balance. It strengthens and stretches out the backs of your legs and increases the flexibility in the ligaments and tendons. It helps to lengthen and straighten the spine.

You can have your baby in a wrap or in the buggy.

Method Hand to Knee Pose

1. Come to standing and spread out your toes on one foot, the foot you will be standing on. Either bare foot or inside your shoes. The wider you have your toes, the more balance you will have. Send your gaze forwards slightly and start to pinpoint an object.

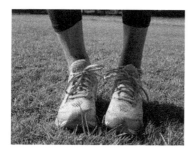

2. Slowly lift one foot off the floor and shift your weight to the standing leg. Engage your quads on the standing leg and engage the core. Bend the lifted knee and hold onto it, wrapping your hands around your shin.

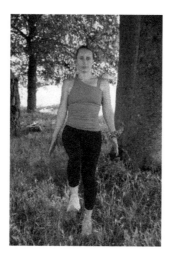 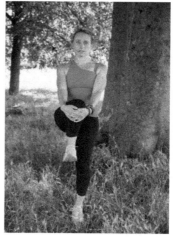

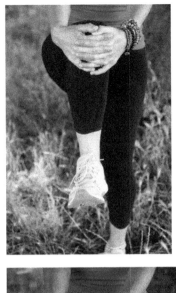

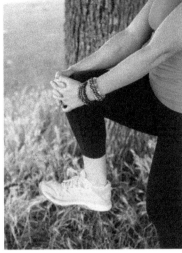

3. Push the heel down towards the floor, flexing the toes.

Correct foot position.

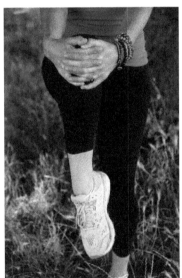

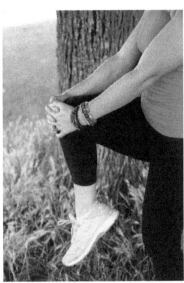

Not correct foot position.

4. Engage your gluteal muscles (buttocks), lift your chest with your tail bone pointing downwards. Lift through the crown of your head, pushing your shoulders down away from your ears and drawing them towards your spine. Pull up your pelvic floor muscles.

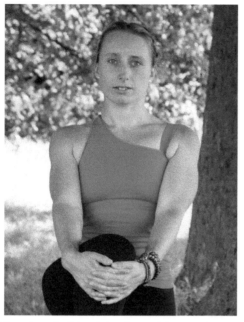

5. With every exhale, draw the knee in closer to your chest, feeling a stretch in the inner groin opening out the hip flexors. Breathe deeply for five breaths.

6. Keeping hold of the leg with one hand, bring the other hand to place it onto your hip. Slowly move the bent knee outwards, keeping the hips centred and squared. This will allow the pelvis to open. Stay here for five breaths.

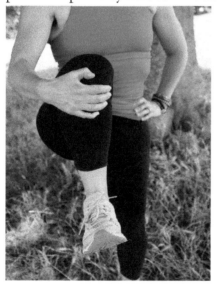

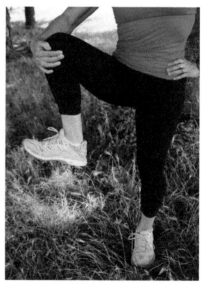

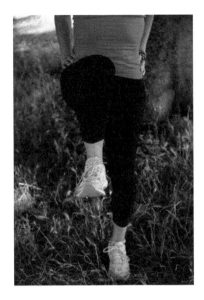 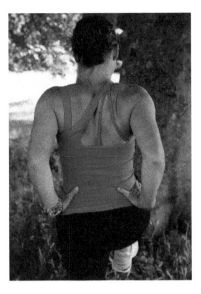

7. Bring the knee back to the centre keeping it lifted still engaging all the leg muscles, bring both hands to wrap around the hips. Bring your elbows backwards drawing the shoulder blades in towards each other.

8. Point your toes slowly straightening the leg. Keep it lifted for one breath and then kick up into the air and lower back down to the floor.

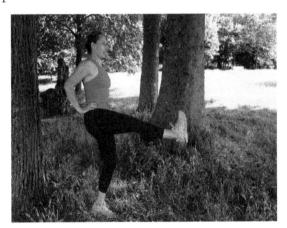 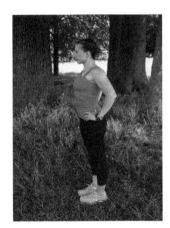

9. This is strong on both legs so shake them out before swapping to the opposite leg.

10. Repeat on the other side.

Tip

Be careful here if you have ankle or lower back problems.

Hold onto the buggy for extra balance if needed.

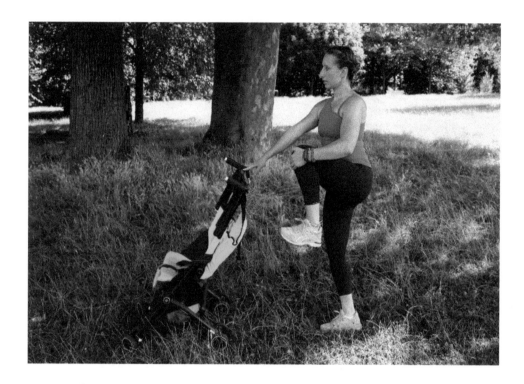

Hold onto the buggy for extra balance if needed.

To move from Knee to Toe Pose, use a strap to create extra length, also try doing it with a bent knee.

Happy Healthy Parents

Make

Happy Healthy Children.' – Relationship, love and happiness

Hand to Big Toe Pose

Method for Hand to Big Toe Pose

1. Follow the instructions on the previous page but instead of holding the knee, hold onto the big toe. Bend the knee and bring your arm inside of the thigh reaching around the outside of the top of the foot. Bring your middle and index finger to wrap around the big toe. Have one hand wrapped around your hips.

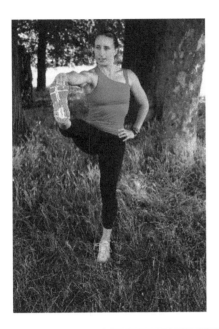
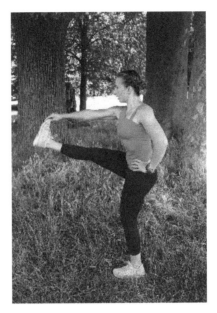

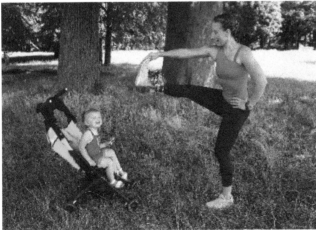

3. Bring back to the front and release the fingers, bringing both hands to the hips. Kick up and back down and shake out both legs.

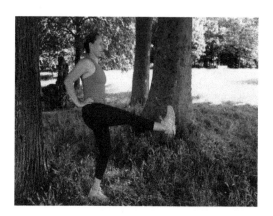
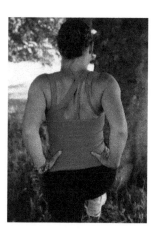

2. Again, bring that foot out to the side keeping form in the hips. Hold for five breaths.

Tip

Hold onto the buggy for extra balance if needed.

To move from Knee to Toe Pose, use a strap to create extra length, also try doing it with a bent knee. If doing Hand to Toe Pose, try having a toy wrapped around your ankle so you can engage play if your baby is in the buggy.

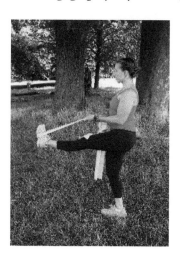
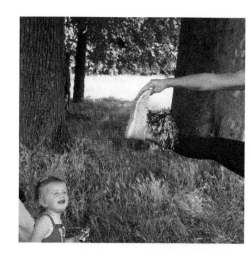

'Sometimes the smallest things take up most room in your heart' – Winnie The Pooh

Low Lunge

Lunges are great for helping target hip flexors and lower spine. The hips can start to tighten once the pregnancy hormones have decreased in the body. Lunges are a great way to keep the hips supple and build strength in the thighs and lower back.

You can have your baby in a wrap close to you or in a buggy. If using a buggy, you can hold onto the handle and push it forwards and backwards to advance the position, also getting a little arm workout too.

Method

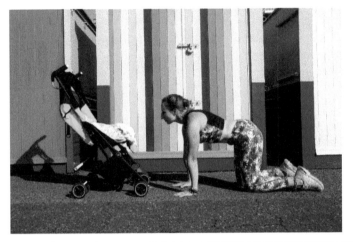

1. Come on to all fours. Have knees stacked under hips. and hands under shoulders.

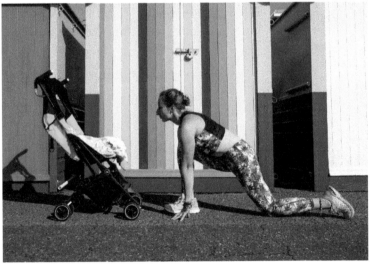

2. Bring one foot in line with your hands, keeping your knee stacked above your ankle. Push forwards slightly to open the lower back and hips.

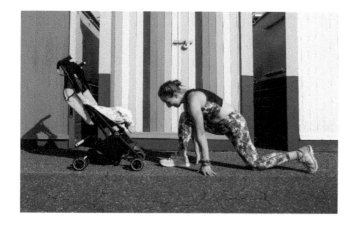

3. Move your other leg backwards slightly keeping your knee on the floor and bring your thigh towards the floor. Press into the front foot, making sure the knee is not folding in on itself. Wrap the inner thigh outwards and look at your big toe. If you cannot see the toe then push the knee out further, keeping an eye on any injuries to the knee or hip area.

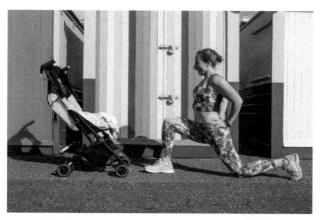

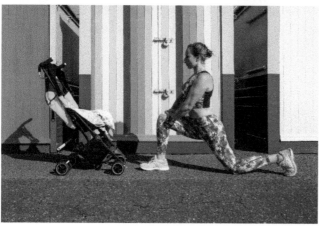

4. Bring your hands to your hips, wrapping them around your waist or place them interlaced onto the top of the thigh.

Page 124 Low Lunge

5. To advance it further bring your arms up above your head, keeping shoulders down away from ears and palms facing towards each other, shoulder width apart or together. Engage your glutes (buttocks) and press down into the ball of the back foot. Engage core and pull pelvic floor muscles up into the abdomen.

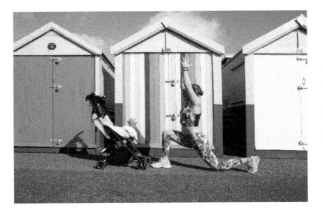

6. Stay here for up to five breaths. Slowly lower down, coming back onto all fours and repeat on the other side.

Tips

Be aware of any serious knee injuries and neck problems. Look down at the floor instead of straight ahead.

If you find you are unbalanced in lunge, move your front foot out towards the side to create a small diagonal invisible line. Another option is to hold onto the buggy for balance.

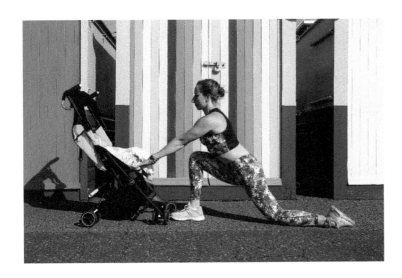

'Lunge? I thought you said Lunch!' – Gym shark

High Lunge and Walking Lunges

Method

Follow the instructions for Low Lunge.

To advance low lunge and come into high lunge push the knee of the back leg backwards. Engage all your leg muscles and glutes, coming onto your toes on the back foot. Push down into the heel, stabilising on the ball of the foot.

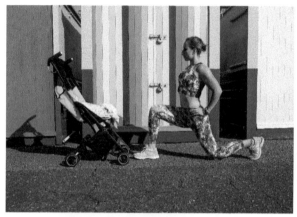
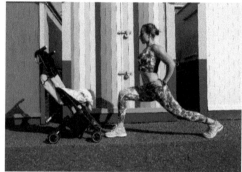

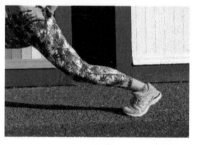

To advance further in Low or High lunge push into the front foot sinking hips down, opening the lower back and on an exhale, bend backwards slightly letting the front of the chest open and bring your arms up. Push the pelvis slightly forward. Keeping shoulders away from ears and relaxing down your back.

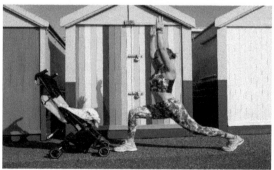

Walking Lunges With a Buggy

1. Come into high lunge, holding onto the handle.

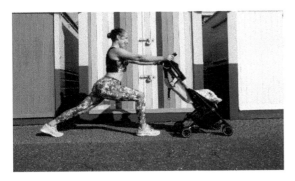

2. Lift the back leg off the floor and walk forwards, landing back into high lunge on that leg. Then move the other leg forward to come into another high lunge. Repeat this walking lunge for 10 to 20 steps.

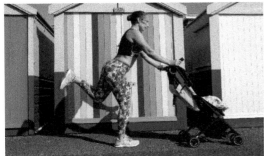
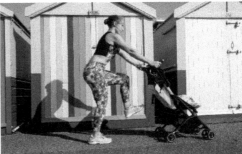

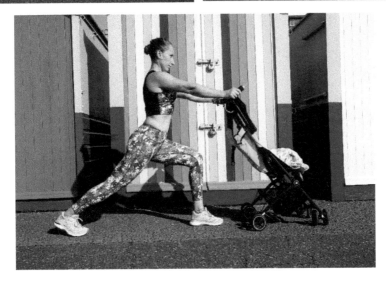

<u>Wall Sit Exercises - with Baby in a Wrap or Using the Buggy</u>

These little wall sits are a killer move as they build strength in the entire legs and lower back. Holding for as long as you can, will then give you different results in different areas of your body. See 'Tips' for different variations with your feet.

<u>Method</u>

Have your baby in a wrap to add more weight to your wall sit or have them on a blanket in front or to the side of you. Even having them in the buggy will help.

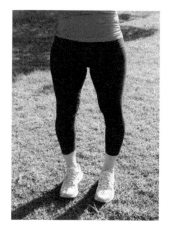

1. Find a wall and place your back against it.

2. Have your knees hip width apart and feet flat onto the floor.

3. Slide down the wall, pushing shoulders into it and activating the core muscles. Bend your knees as you slide down, getting them to a 90-degree angle. Keep your knees tracking over your ankles and no further forwards. Engage your glutes and push the lower back (which normally arches) into the wall.

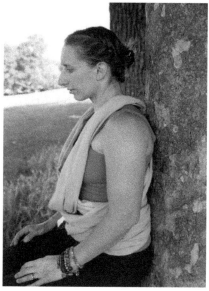

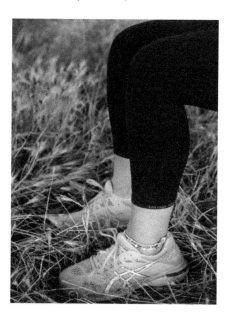

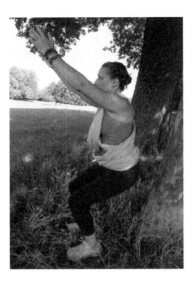

4. Hold for as long as possible, aiming to work up to one to two minutes or even longer.

5. Press into the back of the heels to push out and come back up to standing.

Wall Sit One Legged

Follow the above instructions for wall sit. Once there, keeping core engaged, slowly start to lift one leg off the floor. Hold, then lower and repeat on the other side.

Increase the resistance here by holding baby out in front of you. This will really use your core muscles to help keep you stabilised.

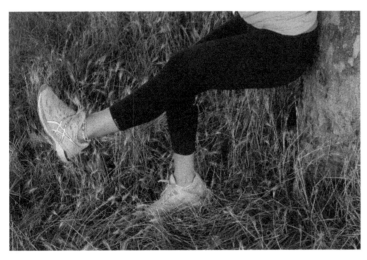 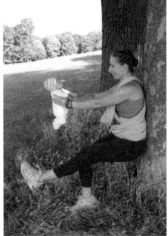

Wall Sit Holding Baby Method

1. Holding your baby, either placing them on your lap to add extra weight or holding them out in front of you with your hands wrapped around their chest, follow the above instructions. Be careful here if baby is not of head holding age, place fingers around the back of his/her head for extra support.

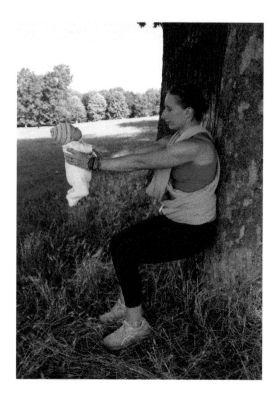
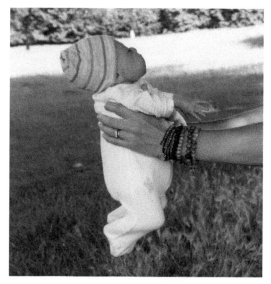

2. If holding baby out in front, keep your shoulders away from your ears and keep the core engaged. This will really work your triceps and bicep muscles.

Wall Sit with the Buggy

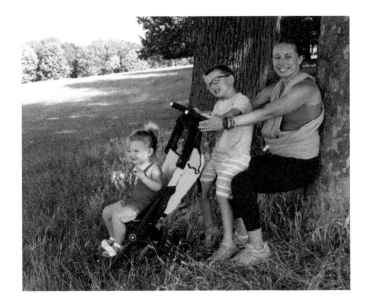

1. Having baby in the buggy, hold onto the handle and assume the position of a wall sit following the above instructions for wall sit.

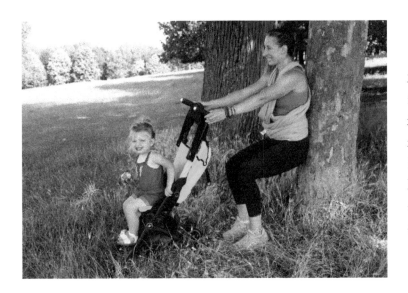

2. Push the buggy away from you and then pull it back it. Keep repeating this exercise for your entire wall sit. Keep shoulders down and away from your ears.

Wall Sit Calf Raises

1. Follow the instructions above for wall sit. Once there, slowly raise both heels off the floor coming onto the toes, stay here for a few breaths and then lower down.

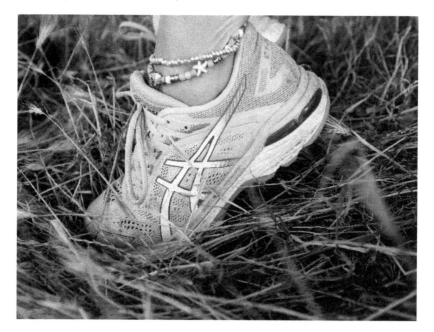

2. Repeat for as long as the hold.

These calf raises will add definition to the lower legs and build strength.

Tip

Pushing into the balls of the feet will activate the quadriceps (quads) while pushing into the heels will activate the glutes and pulling into the heels will activate the hamstrings.

It does not have to be a wall to push up against. It can be the back of a park bench, a tree, a door. Anything with a flat vertical surface will be fine.

'Find the reasons, Lose the excuses,
Gain the results.' - Unknown

Chest Press - Holding Baby and Chest Wall Press

This exercise targets the pectoral muscles (breast muscles), triceps and shoulders. As parents we need the upper body strength to help us through the day with children. Always carrying them around, breast feeding (sorry dads), lifting from the cot and playing with them on the floor. This is a fun exercise to do holding your baby.

Method - Chest Wall Press with Baby in Wrap

1. Come to face a wall being slightly closer than arm's length from it.

2. Have feet hip width apart, toes facing the wall.

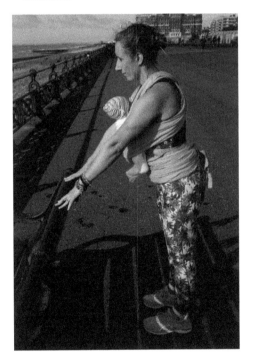

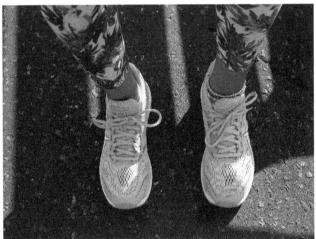

3. Engage quadriceps (quads) by pulling the kneecaps up. Engage your gluteal muscles (buttocks).

4. Bring your weight forward over your toes so your body is about a 45-degree angle to the floor. Have hands resting on the wall about one meter apart. Make sure that baby's head is not touching the wall.

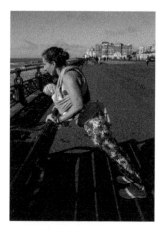

5. Keep leg and arm muscles engaged, slowly push off to bring your arms straight and body parallel with the wall, keeping hands pressed against it.

6. Lower back down to the wall and repeat five to ten times.

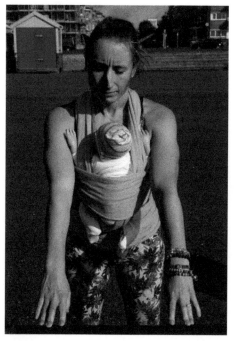 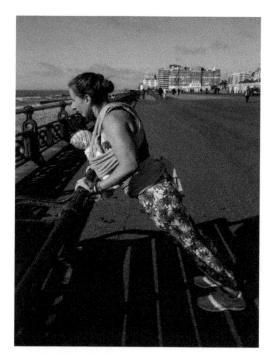

Tip

Only do this exercise with your baby who can hold their own head up.

Try to make silly faces at your baby strengthening the bond between you both.

Method - Chest Press Holding Baby

1. Lay on your back. Either have your knees bent hip width apart or allow your legs to be completely outstretched.

2. Bring your baby to your chest his/her chest facing you.

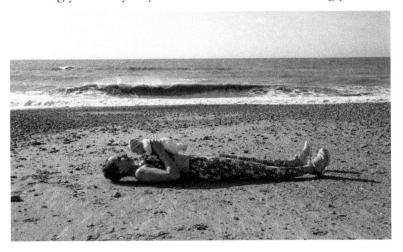

3. Wrap your hands around baby's chest so you are both comfortable.

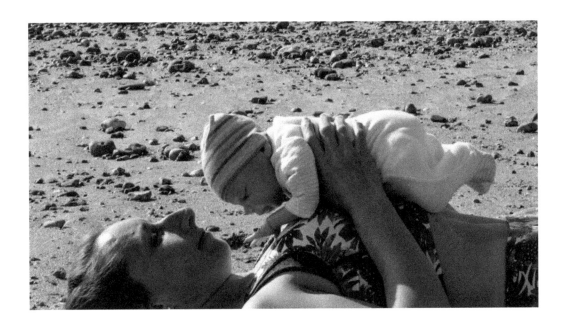

4. Engage your core and arm muscles. Push the shoulder blades into the floor away from your spine. Bring your chin slightly towards your chest, lengthening through your spine.

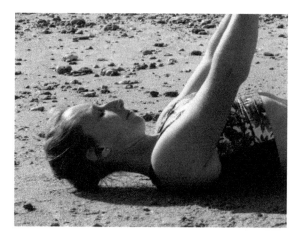

5. Lift your baby from your chest pushing upwards, straightening out your arms but not locking out the elbows. Try to stack your wrists over the shoulders or go as far as you are happy to without hurting shoulders or wrists. Keep your head and shoulders pushed down into the floor.

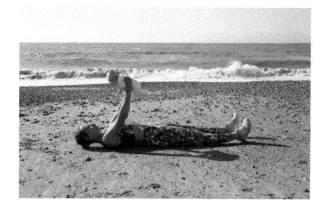

Tip

Make sure your baby has not eaten before doing this exercise. You may be vomited on!

If you have neck problems, rest your head on a pillow.

I almost gave up on my exercise but then I realised who was watching. My baby.
- Gymaholic

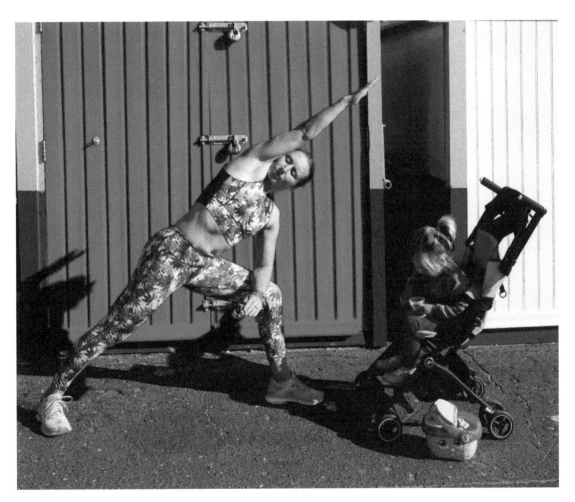

Figure 3 - Side Angle Pose

Chapter Six

Exercises and Yoga Poses using the buggy

Warrior Three Push Outs

Warrior Two Pose

Dancer Pose

Triangle Pose

Side Angle Stretch

Downward Dog to Plank

Plank Variations

Push Up Variations

Squat Variations

Burpee and Burpee Tuck Up's

Tuck Jumps

Bow Pose

Kneeling Superman's

Seated Spinal Twist

Warrior Three Push Outs

Warrior Three strengthens the whole back of the body, including shoulders, hamstrings, calves, ankles, and back. It also tones and strengthens the abdominal muscles. It improves balance, posture, and full-body coordination.

You can have your baby in a wrap or in a buggy for this exercise.

Method

1. Come into mountain pose (see page 35) and then step one leg back coming onto your toes on your back foot and then landing into High Lunge. See page 125 for instructions on High Lunge. Either hold onto the buggy handles or bring arms up above your head,

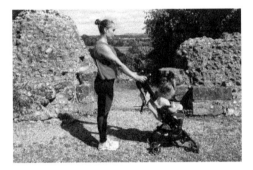

2. Push into your back foot, sending heel down towards the floor, spreading out your toes onto the floor with your front foot engaging all leg muscles. Also engaging the core muscles.

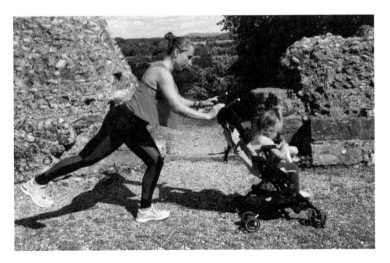

3. As you exhale start to straighten your front leg, bringing your back leg off the mat or floor, lifting it behind you. Engaging your quadriceps (quads) and gluteal muscles (glutes) at the same time.

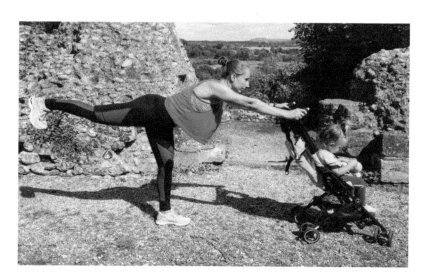

4. From here bring your arms forward so your triceps are facing down parallel with the floor, reaching through your fingertips. Try to get your torso, arms, and back leg all in a straight line. Keep your pelvis centred and pushed back. Stay here for 5-10 breaths, slowly release giving your standing leg a shake out and repeat on the other side.

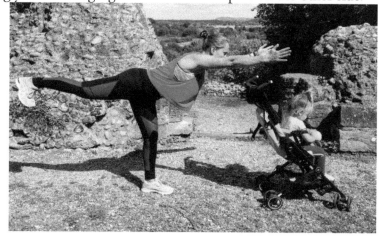

Tip

Be careful in this pose if you have high blood pressure if it is not already under control.

If having your baby in a wrap you may need to support his/her head with one hand as you fold forwards.

If you are finding it hard to balance in Warrior three then hold onto the buggy giving you extra support.

If using the buggy, hold onto the handle with the buggy out in front of you. Repeat the above instructions and when you fold forward bring the buggy backwards and forwards. Tuck your elbows in on the pull towards you. Repeat these five to ten times.

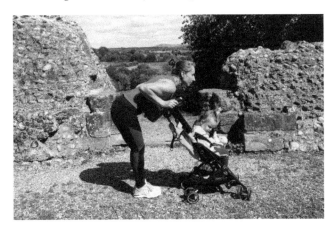

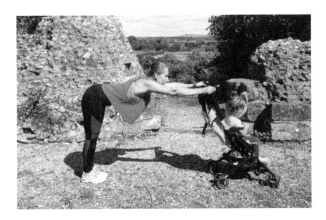

When you arise in the morning. Think of what a precious privilege it is to be alive – to breathe. To think. To enjoy. To love. – Marcus Aurelius

Page 141 Warrior Three

Warrior Two Pose

This strengthens the legs, opens the hips and chest. Warrior Two develops concentration and balance which helps battle internal weakness. It also improves circulation and respiration and energizes the entire body. As parents we need a little energising every now and again.

You can have your baby in a wrap or placed in the buggy.

Method

1. Have your feet about a metre apart and turn the right foot to face forwards and the left foot about 15 degrees inwards. Have heels in line with each other.

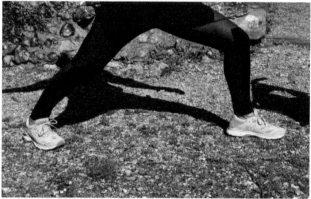

2. Bend your right knee, stacking it over your ankle. Engage your quads and hamstrings and push out the front knee so you can see your big toe. Try to wrap your inner thighs outwards.

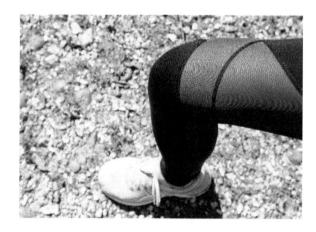

3. Turn your hips and shoulders towards the front and have your arms outstretched. Your right arm in front and your left arm behind you. Turn your head and look at the right middle finger. Making sure that your left arm is not sinking down, engage your arm muscles.

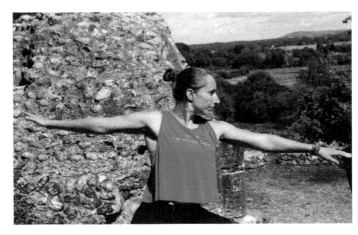

4. Lift shoulders up and draw them backwards, sliding them down your back away from your ears. Press your chest forwards. Keep hips in line with shoulders.

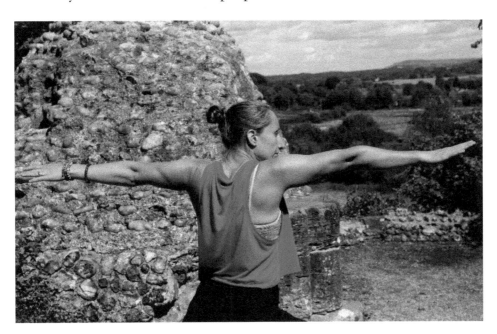

5. Press into your feet, keeping your legs strong. Roll to the outside of your back foot. Sink your hips down towards the floor, with tail bone tucked under. Reach the crown of your head up to lengthen through the spine.

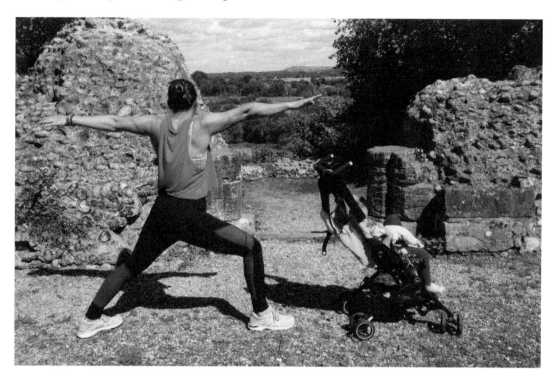

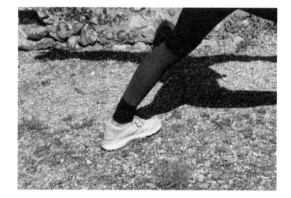

Roll to the outside of your back foot.

6. Breathe and hold for three to six breaths.

7. To release: straighten your legs and turn your feet forward, coming back into Mountain Pose.

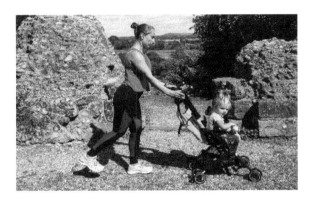 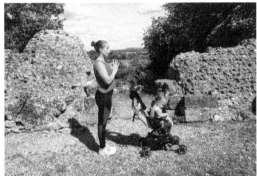

Tips

Be careful in this pose if you have high blood pressure if it is not already under control.

Using a buggy, repeat the instructions but holding the handle in front or to the side, push and pull the buggy backwards and forwards, keeping the front knee bent and in the correct alignment.

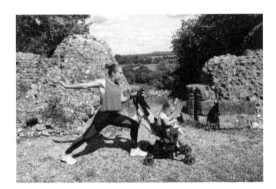 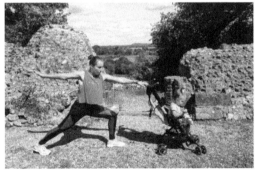

'Be a Warrior, not a Worrier.' Unknown

Dancer Pose and Buggy Version

Dancer Pose builds full body strength, flexibility, and coordination. It opens the shoulders, chest, and hips, as it stretches and strengthens the thighs, ankles, and abdomen. This pose develops greater flexibility in your spine, shoulders, and hamstrings.

This pose can be done with baby in a wrap or placed in the buggy.

Method

1. Come into Mountain Pose (see page 35) and shift your weight onto one foot, spreading out your toes as you go.

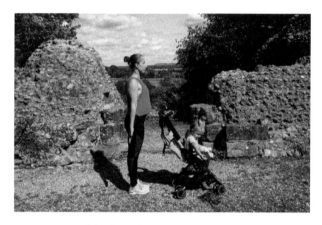

2. Start to lift the other leg off the floor, bending your knee and bringing the heel of your foot up and backwards. Lift your kneecap up on your standing leg engaging your quads.

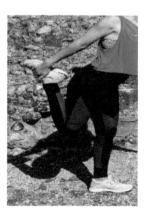

3. Reach back with the same arm to grab your heel or ankle, lifting your torso and pelvic floor at the same time and pushing your tailbone down and under.

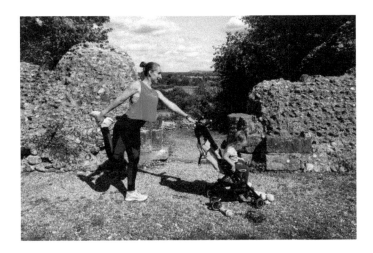

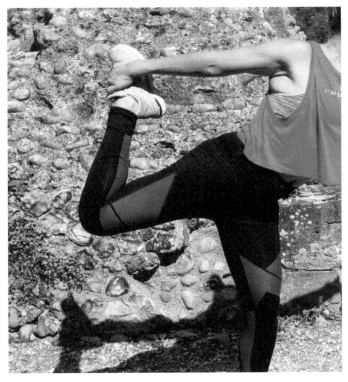

4. Extend your thigh parallel with the floor, pushing your foot into your hand.

5. Stretch your other arm forward parallel to the floor, still slightly lifting your torso but bringing it slightly folded forwards.

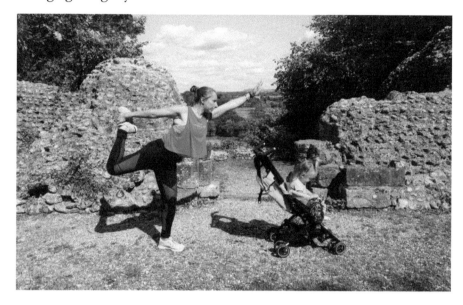

6. Stay here for 30 seconds to a minute and then release back down.

Tip

For balance use the buggy. Hold onto the handle with your outstretched arm. For a more advanced version push the buggy back and forth, engaging the arm muscles. To advance this further push the buggy so your chest is parallel to the floor. Engage the leg muscles to push back up and repeat five to ten times then swap legs.

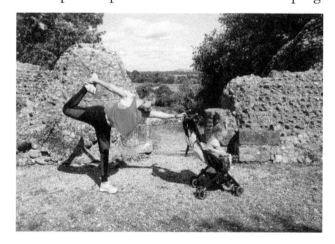

'Strength doesn't come from what you do. It comes from doing what you thought you couldn't do.' – Simple reminders

Triangle Pose Using a Buggy

Triangle Pose is a therapeutic pose that provides many benefits including strengthening of the core and legs. It improves digestion and stimulates the abdominal organs.

Use the buggy for this exercise for different variations. You can hold a toy in one hand and use it to play with your child when you are reaching over. This is great fun for the baby.

Method

1. Position the buggy next to the front foot. Stand with your feet about four feet apart.

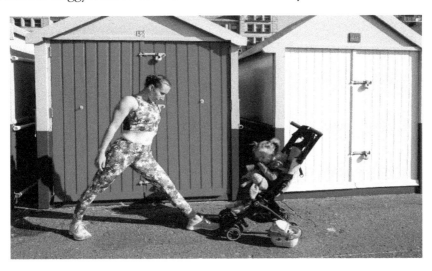

2. Turn your left foot out about 90 degrees and your right foot about 15 degrees.

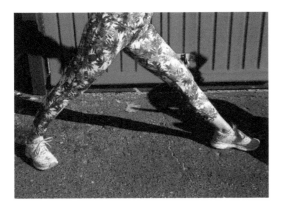

3. Have your arms outstretched and look down your left arm.

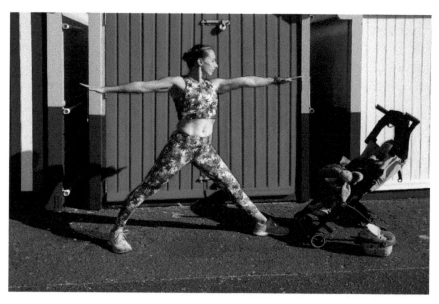

4. Engage your quadriceps by bringing your kneecaps up. Rotate the inner thigh up on the front leg while rolling onto the outside of the back foot, keeping an arch in the foot. Pull pelvic floor muscles up into the abdomen.

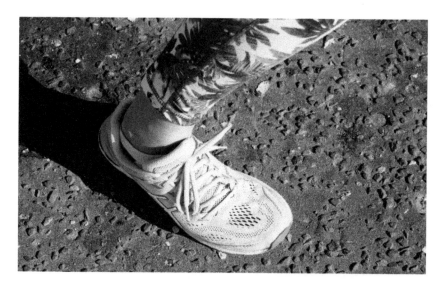

5. On an exhale, reach as far forward as you can before folding down over your left leg, placing your hand on the bar of the buggy or the footplate. Send your hips backwards as you fold down, engaging the core.

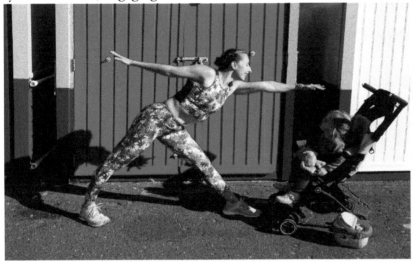

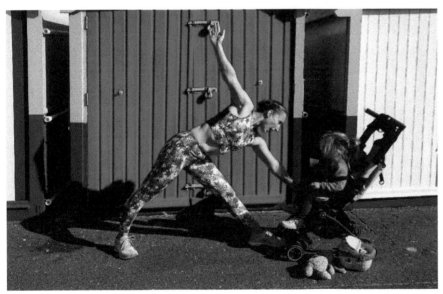

6. Bring your right arm up so your hand is stacked above your shoulder. Draw your shoulder blades towards each other, chest lifted. Send your gaze to look up at your outstretched right arm. Try not to arch your torso and keep your legs straight.

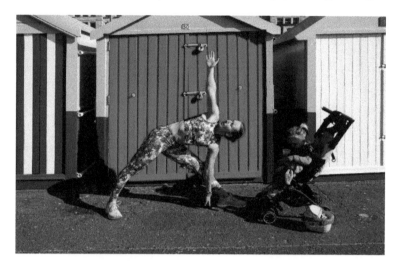

7. To come out, keep legs engaged and lift trough your torso releasing back to the start position. Repeat on the right side.

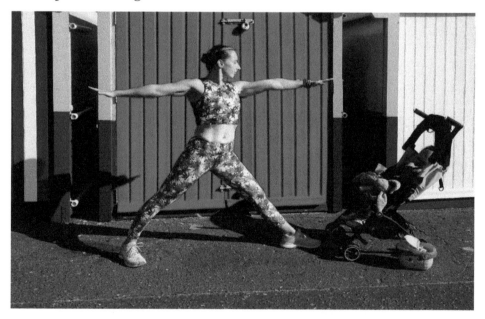

Tips

To advance Triangle, try to push the buggy back and forth with the lower hand, keeping all muscles engaged.

Be aware in this exercise if you have low blood pressure.

Neck Problems (do not turn your head, just look straight ahead).

Heart conditions (practice against a wall or bench for extra stability and keep top arm by your hip).

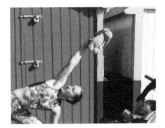

Hold a toy in the arm which is lifted and try to distract your baby. This will engage play with them.

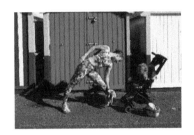

If you suffer with high blood pressure (turn your head to look down when in the full pose and bring your top arm down).

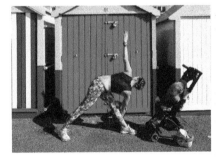

A slight twist on this variation will be to twist this triangle. From instruction six once you are in Triangle, drop the top arm down and place that hand onto the outside of the front foot, twisting through the spine. Keep your legs engaged and send your hips backwards. The bottom hand will then come up back behind you, creating a twist the other way. Send your gaze over the other shoulder looking up. A block, bench or the buggy may be of use here to get the height in the twist.

'If you listen to your body when it whispers, you won't have to hear it scream.' Unknown

Page 153 Triangle

Side Angle Stretch

This pose strengthens and stretches your legs, knees, and ankles. It also stretches your hip flexors, spine, waist, chest and lungs, and shoulders. It stimulates your abdominal organs and increases stamina.

Baby can either be in a wrap, but you will probably need to support his/her head, or they can be in the buggy. There are three options here for this pose.

Method

1. From Mountain Pose, have your feet wide about your leg length apart.

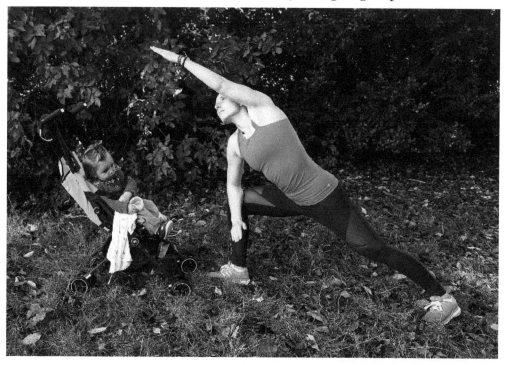

2. Move your left foot out about 90 degrees and turn your right foot to face the front of the mat. Bend the front knee, making sure that the knee is directly over the ankle. Aim to get the underside of the thigh parallel to the floor. Aim to have both heels in line with each other. Engage the leg muscles. Make sure the right knee is not folding in on itself and engage the inner thigh to rotate it outwards slightly.

3. Bring your arms out to the sides parallel to the floor, palms facing downwards. Pick up the shoulders and slide them down the back. Bend the front arm to come down on to the top of the bent knee.

4. With the other hand, bring it up and over your head, brushing past the ear, palms facing towards the floor. Lengthen all the way down the body. Aim to have hand, shoulder, hips, knees, and ankles all in a straight line.

5. Roll onto the outside of the back foot, pressing heels down.

6. Look up at the raised hand or underneath the armpit opening out your chest.

7. Stay here for five to ten breaths. Release by pushing into both feet and repeat on the other side.

Tip

Be careful if you have neck problems here. Do not turn your head to look up at the palm of the hand. Look straight ahead or down to the floor.

Have a toy in the raised arm and move it around to keep baby amused. It will also be fun for you.

Different variations here are to bring the right arm down towards the floor, resting the palm of the hand on the floor. If it does not reach you can add a block or the buggy foot plate. Try to open more in the chest, pushing slightly in towards the inner thigh.

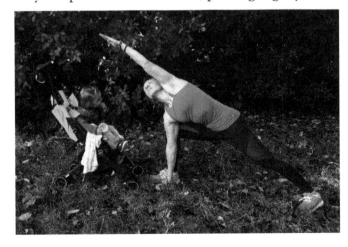

Another variation is to bring your right arm underneath the thigh and have your palm facing upwards. Bring the left arm behind you and try to grasp both hands together. Use a band or strap if necessary.

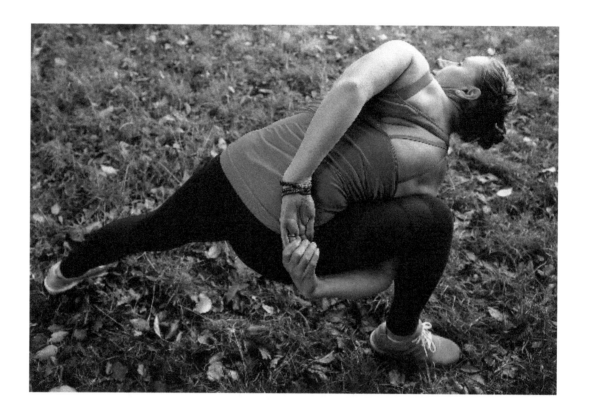

'It is your duty to keep your body in good health. Without health, it is impossible to keep a clear and strong mind.' - *Buddha*

Calf Raises

These are fantastic to build up strength in your calves as well as to stretch out your lower leg muscles.

There are two variations here: calf raises holding onto buggy handle and walking calf raises.

Have your baby in a wrap here or in the buggy.

Method

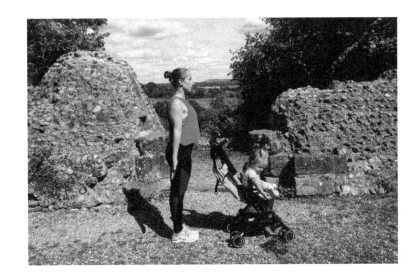

1. Stand up straight with feet hip width apart. Engage your core and push into the balls of your feet.

2. Hold onto the buggy handle for balance and slowly start to come up onto your toes.

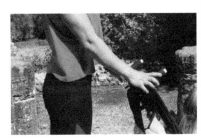 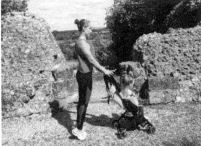

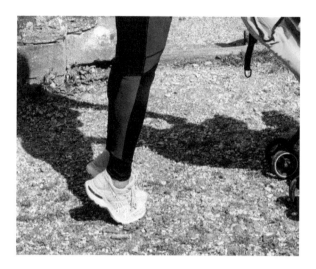

3. Lower back down and repeat for 10 to 20 lifts.

Calf Raise Walks

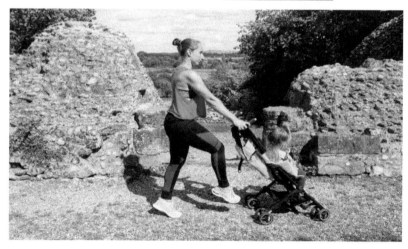

1. Follow the instructions above, when up on toes, lift one leg forward to do one pace.

2. Lower back down and then swap to the other leg bringing that forward and come up onto toes. Lower back down.

3. Keep your strides normal but try to come up high onto your toes.

Tip

An advanced version is to push one foot behind you lifting it off the floor and using the other foot to come up to do calf raises. Do 10 to 20 lifts on one leg and swap sides.

These are a great exercise to do anywhere. Maybe try doing them while waiting in a queue or while you are cleaning your teeth.

Be careful here if you have torn the Achilles tendon or the calf muscle. These exercises are great to build up strength and work on building muscles in the lower leg area.

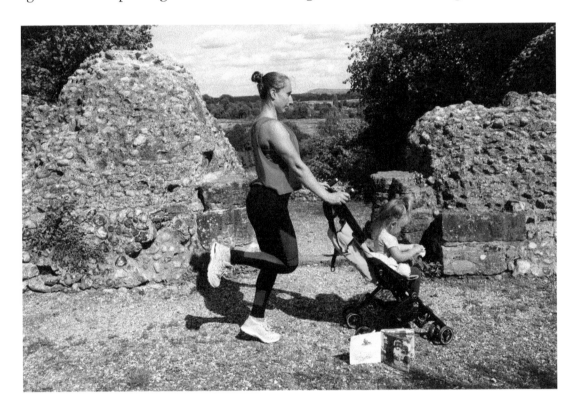

'It takes four weeks for you to notice your body changing,
Eight weeks for your friends and 12 weeks for the rest of the world.
Give it 12 weeks. Don't Quit.' - Nike

Downward Facing Dog to Plank Walk Outs

Downward Facing Dog is such an energising pose. It builds up strength in the upper arms and gives you space and opening in the back, neck, chest, hips and shoulders. We as parents need energy most of the day to look after our little ones. This energises all muscles and rejuvenates the oxygen flow around the body in the blood stream to help your feel more alive.

Method

1. Come onto the floor into Tabletop position having your hands slightly forward of your shoulders and your knees underneath your hips, keeping knees hip distance apart. Tuck your toes under.

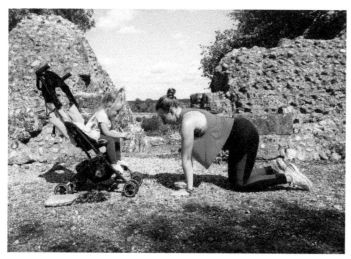 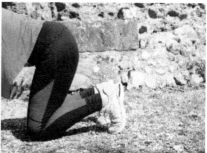

2. Push hands away from the floor and relax your upper back between the shoulder blades. Wrap your triceps under to firm the shoulder blades down your back.

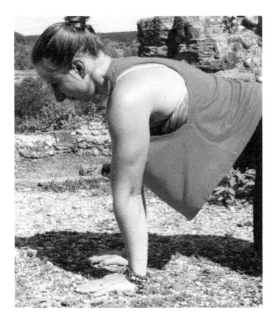

3. Spread your fingers wide and push through the thumb and index finger, trying to create a small dome in the palm of your hands.

4. Exhale, lift your knees and draw your spine backwards from your pelvis, so that your arms and back form one line. Lifting your hips towards the sky, tailbone lifting towards the sky, pushing heels down towards the floor.

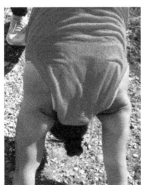 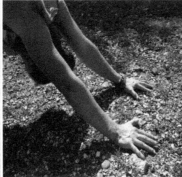 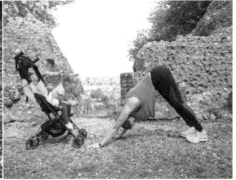

5. Engage your quads (quadriceps) by drawing the knees up into thighs. Pull the pelvic floor muscles up into the abdomen and engage the core muscles.

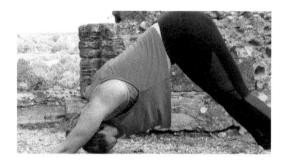

6. Gaze up to your thighs, keeping your head in line with the arms. With every exhale try to push your chest further towards your thighs. Keep the lift in the pelvis and heels pushing down towards the floor.

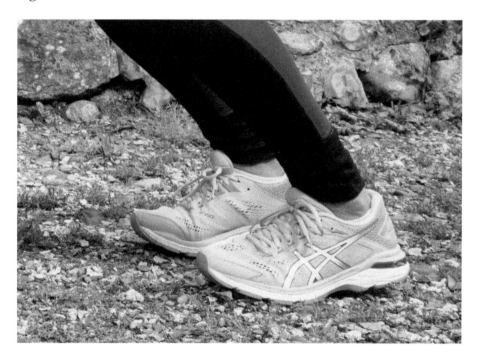

7. Stay here for one minute, breathing deeply into the chest, melting it towards the floor.

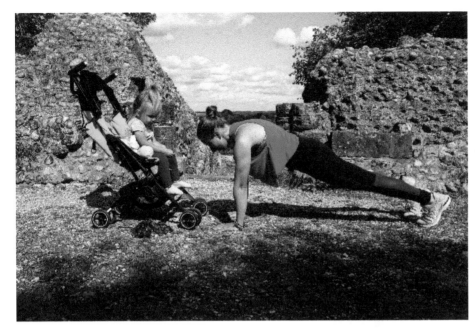

8. From Downward Dog start to walk your hands along the floor, engaging the core coming into High Plank. See page 164 for High plank.

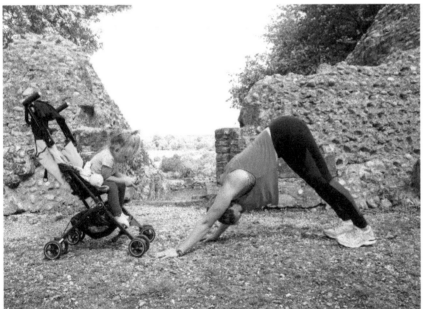

9. From Plank then walk back to Downward Dog, keeping form and all muscles engaged. Repeat five to ten times.

10. To come out, drop down onto knees and come back to a tabletop position.

Tip

Be careful in this pose if you have high blood pressure, suffer with headaches, or Carpal Tunnel Syndrome.

Do not lock out your elbows or knees.

Have the buggy at the end of the Plank position so you can touch the stroller footplate with your hands or say boo to your child. Children love to join in the workout. It also makes it fun.

If this is quite tight on your wrists, then come down to rest on your forearms pushing into the elbows and roll onto the outside of the forearms.

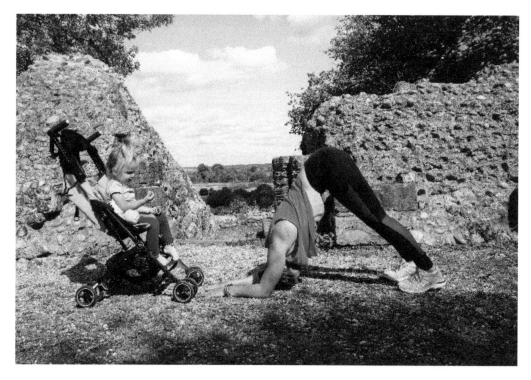

'You will never always be motivated; you have to learned to be disciplined.'- Quote inspire

Plank (Different Varieties)

Plank is a great way to strengthen your arms, wrists, and spine. It tones your abdomen and starts to help burn fat.

Here we are using the traditional Plank but then to advance it further we will be using the buggy for Plank Walk Outs, Plank Pulls, Plank Tucks, Plank Knee to Elbow, Reverse Plank, Reverse Plank Touches and Plank Push Outs.

Have baby in front of you on a pillow or cushion or in the buggy for this exercise.

Children and babies love seeing parents working out as this gives them extra comfort knowing that you are close by. Try making silly faces at them. It makes that bond even stronger and passes the time while in Plank.

Plank Method

1. Have your hands shoulder width apart and spread the fingers to distribute the weight evenly throughout the hands and feet. Slightly turn the upper arms inwards engaging the triceps.

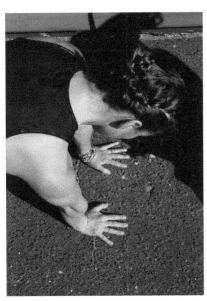 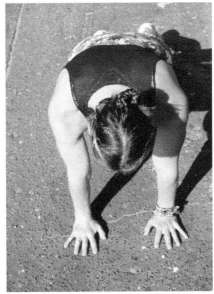

2. Engage the shoulders by pushing up through the chest and drawing the shoulder blades away from the spine.

3. Engage your core, straightening out your legs, pushing the weight through to the feet.

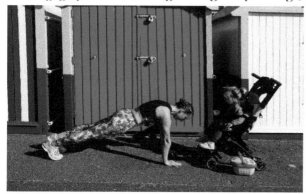 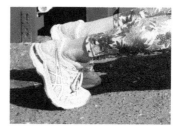

4. Bring the kneecaps up into the quadriceps (quads) to engage the legs, keeping the pelvis lifted. You are aiming to get shoulders, hips, knees, and feet all in a straight line.

5. Try to push your heels down towards the floor.

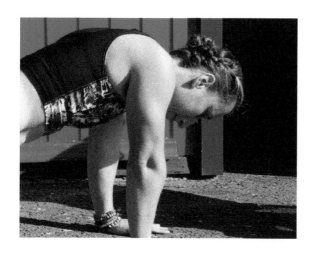

6. Send you gaze through to the floor. Imagine holding a tennis ball in between your chin and chest. This will help keep your spine in the correct alignment.

7. Plank pose is not about repetitions; it is about keeping the correct form for a set amount of time. Set your time and then repeat five or six sets, aiming to increase the time gradually but keeping form. Aim for around 15 seconds to start with. (For a gentler version which is on knees see the Tips section).

Plank Walkouts

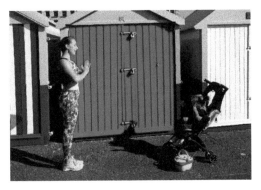

1. Start from standing and then fold forward with your hands towards the floor, crouching down and the head facing forwards, lifting through the pelvis. Engage your core and quads and slowly start to bend at the knees.

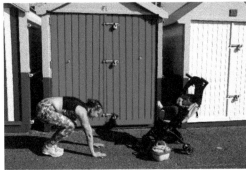

2. Walk your hands forwards until your get to a Plank position. Do not allow your body to arch down, keeping your shoulders pressed outwards away from your spine. Hold for two breaths and then, keeping your core engaged, walk your hands back to the start position.

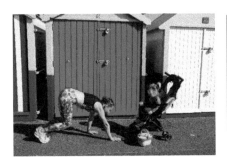
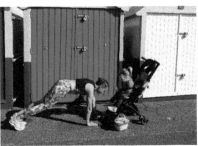

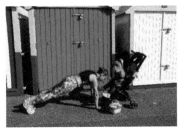

3. Repeat five to ten times.

To advance this pose hold the foot plate of the buggy with your hands and either coming onto knees or plank position, engage your core, pushing the buggy away from you and bring it back to the centre again. Try this for five rounds. This will really fire up your core.

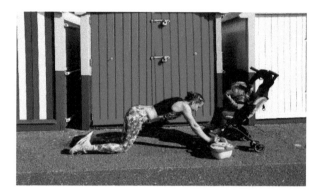

Onto knees and slowly push out.

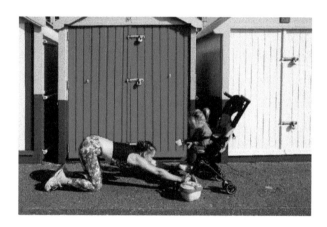

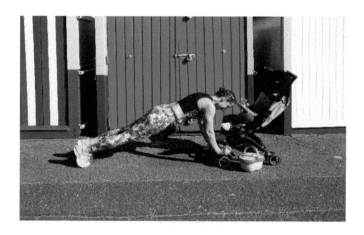

Plank legs straight.

Page 168 Plank Walkouts

Plank Tucks Using the Buggy

1. Bring the tops of your feet to the foot plate and follow the instructions above to get into full Plank position.

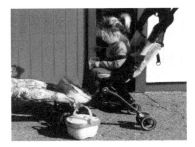 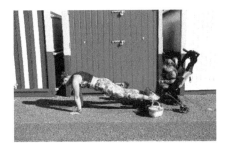

2. Keeping your core engaged and pelvic floor muscles engaged, start to draw your knees in towards your chest, lengthening through your tail bone and pushing through your shoulders.

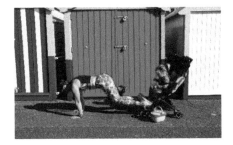 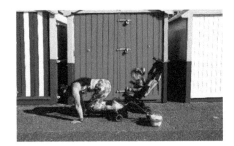

3. Push your legs away again to come back to Plank. Repeat five to ten times.

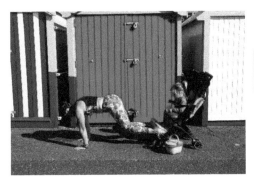 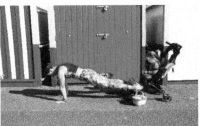

Reverse Plank

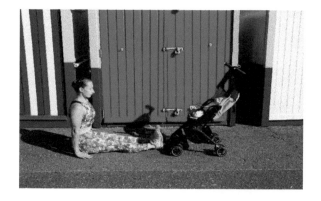

1. Come onto the floor in a seated position with legs in front out straight.

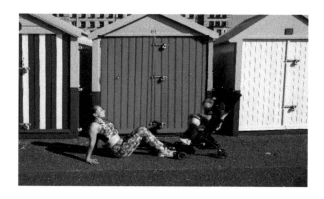

2. Bring your arms slightly behind you, palms to the floor and fingers pointing towards you, bending slightly through the elbows, and keeping knees bent.

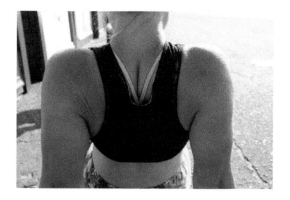

3. Draw your shoulder blades towards each other and lift through the chest.

4. Engaging your glutes, core, and quads, slowly lift the front of your pelvis off the floor, pressing down into the heels aiming to get toes to touch the floor.

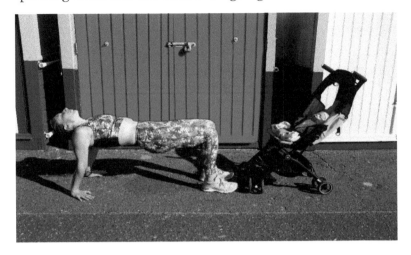

5. Imagine a piece of string attached to your pelvis trying to lift you up.

6. Stay here for ten seconds, aiming to do three rounds of ten seconds. Slowly lower back down and release.

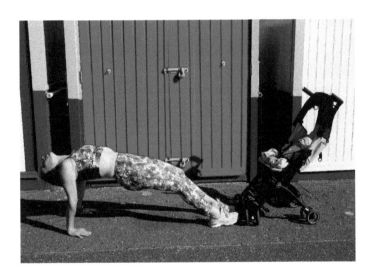

To increase the stretch, have your legs out straight.

Reverse Plank Touches with a Buggy

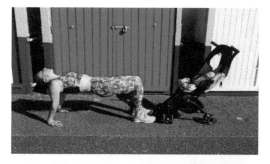

1. See above for reverse Plank

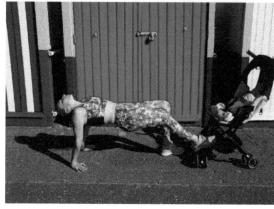

2. From the Lifted Reverse Plank position touch one foot onto the foot plate of the buggy.

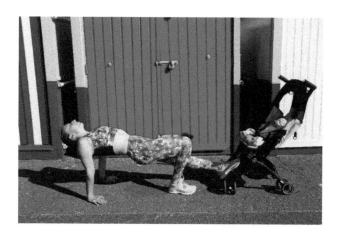

3. Slowly lower that leg and repeat on the other side.

4. Aim to do three rounds of ten seconds.

Plank Pull Using a Buggy

1. Start in Plank position from the above instructions. With the tops of your toes, place them on the foot plate of the buggy. Engage your core, quads, and glutes. Again, push up through your chest drawing shoulder blades away from the spine.

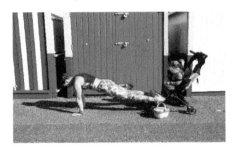 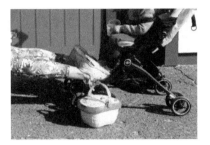

2. Start to move your hands pulling your body and the buggy forwards for five to ten strides with your arms. Keep your core engaged and legs strong.

3. Reverse the walk and slowly drop knees to floor bringing your feet off the foot plate.

Tips For Planks

Check if you have Diastasis Recti. (See page 13) You can still do Planks, but you will need to be supported either staying on your knees or using a raised surface, for example a bench or the foot plate of the buggy but stay on your knees.

Do not do if you have Carpel Tunnel Syndrome.

Try not to hold your breath in any of the Plank positions.

Be aware of any wrist problems. Lower down onto forearms and follow the same instructions as above.

To advance Plank, try drawing your hands towards your toes and your toes towards your hands, always engaging the core. This will really fire up the core muscles all the way around your middle.

Do not look up in Plank position. This will increase the strain in your neck and spine and will send your Plank position out of alignment. Keep your gaze towards the floor in between your hands.

Plank Knee to Elbow Advancing it Using a Buggy or Bench

1. Once we have got the correct Plank position, we can then move onto advancing it to Plank Knee to Elbow.

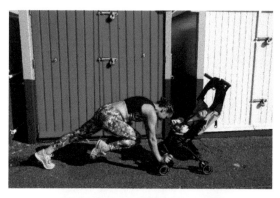

2. From Plank, keeping core engaged, lift the right leg off the floor bending at the knee and draw it inwards towards your chest aiming to touch your elbow. Keep your foot up away from the floor. Push back to the start position. Repeat on the left leg. Do these 10 to 15 times with each leg.

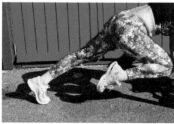

3. To advance it, place your feet onto the footplate of the buggy or use a bench to add height. Repeat the instructions as above.

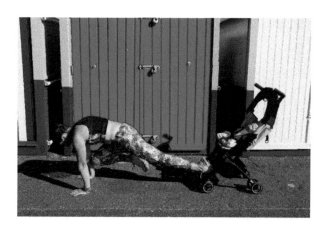

Page 174 Plank Knee to Elbow

Plank Push Outs

Be careful here if your Diastasis Recti has not completely healed. I would probably not recommend this exercise until it has completely rectified itself.

1. Have the buggy in front of you, coming onto all fours, having hands stacked under shoulders and knees stacked under hips. Holding onto the footplate, engaging your core slowly start to roll out until your torso is around a 45-degree angle. Engage your quads here and push shoulders down away from your ears.

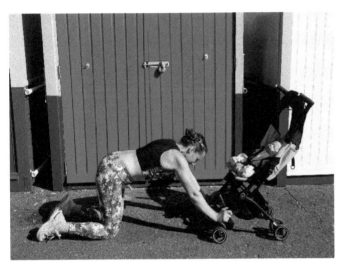

2. Hold and then reverse coming back to the start position. Repeat five to ten times.

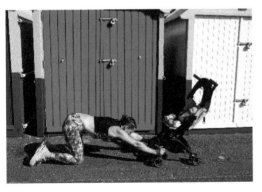

'Here's to you
'Bouncing Forward'
after having your babies,
and helping your already amazing body
to heal as it should and get to
where you want it to be.
Only you get to decide that.' - Unknown

Push-Up Variations

Push-ups are a great little exercise to add into any routine. They use your entire muscles to help stabilise you while doing a push up. This exercise also improves overall strength and stretches out the back and arm muscles. It helps to burn fat and delivers more oxygen around the body as most of the major muscle groups are being used. Muscles need oxygen to recover. This exercise can help prevent shoulder injuries due to the amount of muscle being used in the upper body. It also prevents lower back problems

The different variations here are push-ups, decline push-up, one legged decline push-up and incline push-up.

Have your baby on a cushion or blanket here or in the buggy.

Method

1. Come onto all fours with your hands slightly wider than shoulder width apart but in line with your shoulders and your knees stacked under hips. Have your fingers pointing away from you or if it is quite stressful on the wrists then draw hands in slightly.

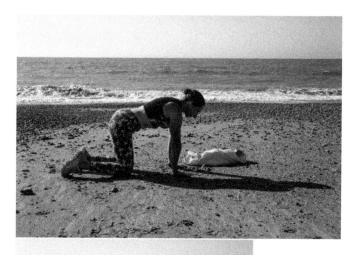

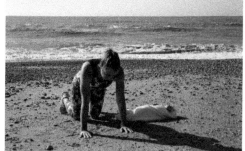

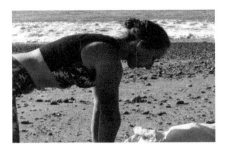

2. Keep your gaze slightly forwards just past your hands.

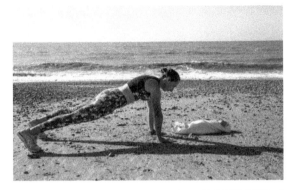

3. Engage your core and gluteal muscles (glutes) and push your feet backwards having them slightly wider than hip width apart. The further you have them apart, the easier it will be for you to balance. You are aiming for your body to be straight line like Plank Pose. Starting from your head, to shoulders, hips, knees, and ankles.

4. Slowly start to lower your body down, bending at the elbows to form a 90-degree angle. You can go lower if you wish. Maybe try to lower down to touch the floor with your chest. Make sure that your elbows are slightly in towards your chest. Elbows pushing out will put extra strain on them and will cause injury.

5. Push up to come back to the start, ending with elbows straight but not locked out. Repeat for as many as you wish but keep your form correct. As soon as you feel your arms are pushing out then stop and repeat at a later stage. This will give your arms a chance to rest.

An easier version is to come onto knees and follow the above instructions.

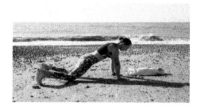 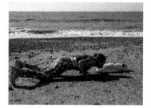

Decline Push-Up Method

Using the buggy, have your feet placed onto the footplate just about more than hip width apart. Repeat instructions for normal push-up.

One Legged Decline Push-Up Method

1. The same as above but only place one foot onto the footplate of the buggy. Have the other foot hovering by the side of the buggy. This will fire up your core immensely.

2. Repeat the instructions above.

Incline Push-Up Method

1. Using the buggy and having the brake off, place hands on the footplate and from here do a push-up following the above instructions.

2. This one will be quite unstable as the buggy will be moving so you'll need to engage your core and glutes tight to keep the buggy in one place.

Tips

Be aware of any shoulder pain, poor posture in this pose and excessive weight (too heavy to lift safely) in this exercise.

Start on knees if this is easier and build up to a full push-up as you build strength in your upper body.

Try drawing your toes towards your hands and hands towards your toes. This will fully engage your core. Try pushing your heels down towards the floor as this will lengthen the calf muscles.

'You don't know your limits until you PUSH YOURSELF past them.' – Robin Sharma

Squat Variations

Squats help to build up your entire leg muscles and create a metabolic response, breaking down fats and building up muscle in your entire body. They target mobility and balance which will help you with everyday activities, especially changing your baby's nappy while squatting on the floor (which I do a lot of). Squats will also build strong stable legs for extra stability.

People are quite afraid to do squats because of all the hype around being bad for your knees, but if done correctly they improve knee stability and strengthen the muscles all around the knee.

Squats are amazing at creating that perfect shaped bottom.

The squats illustrated here are squat, squat chest push outs holding baby, squat push outs with buggy and squat walk.

There are different options here to have your baby in. When doing a normal squat, either have your baby in the buggy or by your side on a pillow or blanket or wearing in a wrap. For the other squats, your baby can be in the buggy.

Squat Method

1. Come into a standing position with your feet slightly wider than your hips. Turn your toes slightly outward, heels slightly inward.

2. Engage the thighs and rotate the inner thighs outwards slightly.

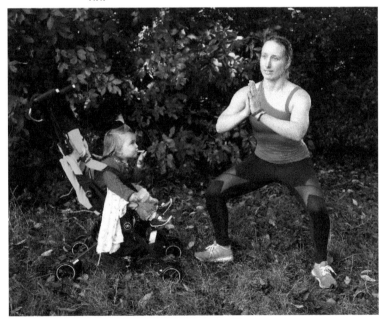

3. Bring your hands to your hips or out in front of you.

4. Engage your core, pulling pelvic floor muscles up and slightly push the weight into the back of the heels.

5. Start to slowly bend your knees, lowering your thighs until they are parallel with the floor. Keep the knees hip distance apart, not letting them fold in, as this creates tension in the knee joints.

6. Keep shoulders away from your ears and chest lifted and tail bone facing down towards the floor. Send your gaze forwards and not up or down as this will create tension in the neck area.

7. Keep your spine long. If you want to go further, then lower down a bit more keeping form in the back and knees.

8. Push through your heels to slowly come back up to standing. Repeat five to ten times, less if you have never done them before.

Squat Chest Pushouts Holding Baby Method (make sure baby is of head-holding age)

1. Follow the above instructions, but instead of having your hands around your hips or in prayer position, hold your baby out in front of you.

2. To do this, hold your baby in a safe position holding under their armpits with your hands wrapped around their chest.

3. On your exhale when squatting, bend your elbows and bring baby in towards your chest. Stay here for one breath and then on an inhale, push back up to standing. Repeat these five to ten times.

Squat Push Outs with a Buggy Method

Hold the handle of the buggy in front of you and follow the above instructions for squat chest push outs.

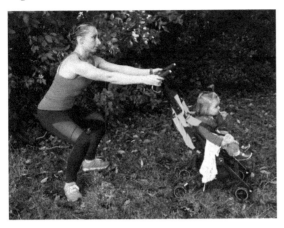

Squat Walk Method

1. Have your baby in the buggy and hold onto the handle.

2. Follow the instructions for 'squat' and get to number seven. From here start to walk around pushing the buggy and keeping form in your lower back and knees. Take eight to ten strides and then come back up to standing, pushing through the back of the heels. This really works the quads and glutes. Start with a lower number of strides if you wish and then build up to ten.

Tip

Squats can be done anywhere. Try squatting while feeding your baby in the highchair. They will find it funny. This will be a great bonding exercise and makes exercise fun for you.

For squat push outs with baby, try making funny faces to really engage with them.

Just be careful in this exercise if you have lower back or knee problems. This will be fine for both if you have the correct form.

'You don't get the ass you want by sitting on it.' - Pintrest

Burpee and Burpee Tuck Ups

This is an amazing set of exercises to burn fat and build up strength all over the body. It is an all body workout which works the arms, back, core, legs and works the cardiovascular system as it increases your heart and respiration rate, working your body harder. Please be careful here if you are still healing with your pelvic floors and if you still have diastasis recti. This exercise is not advised until you are happy you can carry it out correctly or have been signed off by your doctor.

Have your baby in a buggy or on a pillow or blanket next to you.

Burpee Method

1. Come into a standing position having feet hip width apart. Engage your core and slightly bend your knees. Having hands down by your sides, push into the balls of the feet and explode up to jump up into the air swinging arms up over your head.

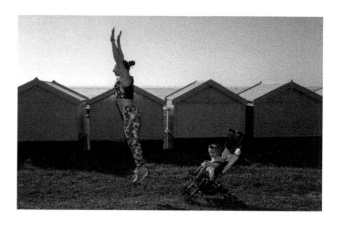

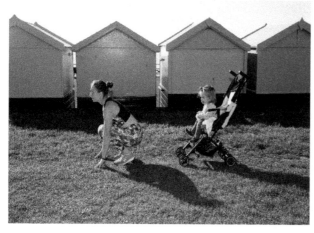

2. As you land, come down into a squat sinking hips lower than your knees, keeping the chest lifted and gazing forward.

3. Place your hands down onto the floor just under your shoulders, spreading out the fingers.

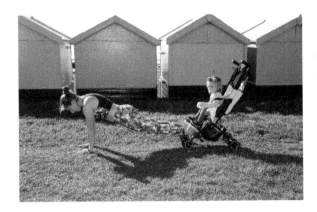

4. Engaging core, step or jump back to a High Plank. (see page 164)

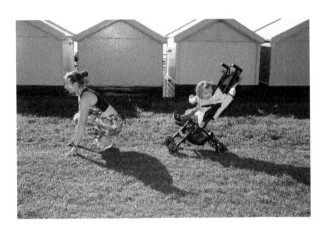

5. From Plank, keeping gluteal muscles (glutes) and quadriceps (quads) engaged, step or jump back to a squat. Having hands placed onto the floor, fingers spread out.

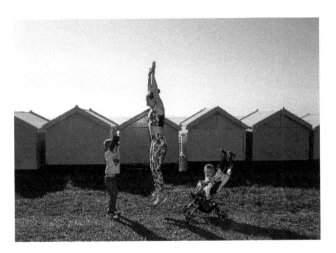

6. Pushing into the heels, explode up to a jump, bending knees and coming off the floor. As you land, bend knees slightly to soften the impact on the knees. Come back to a standing position. This is one whole repetition (rep). Repeat as many times as you would like, aiming for five to ten reps.

Burpee Tuck up Method Using a Buggy

Follow the instructions as above and when you come to High Plank place the tops of your feet onto the foot plate of the buggy. Engaging your core and glutes, draw in your knees towards your chest, then push back to a plank. Keep form in the shoulders drawing the shoulder blades away from each other and not collapsing in the chest. Do one rep, then place feet back onto the floor getting back onto Plank.

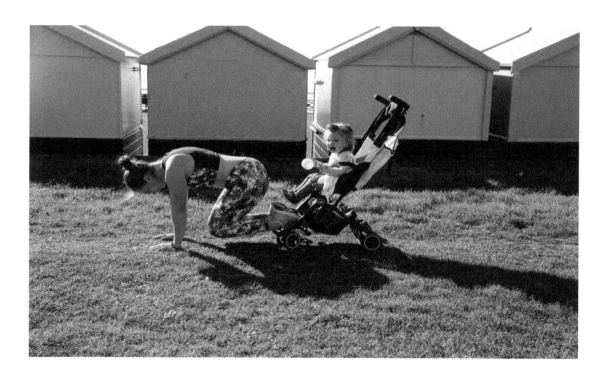

'Fitness is not about being better than someone else...

It's about being better than you used to be.' – Inspirational quotes

Tuck Jump Variations

These little jumps are amazing at burning fat. They activate your core, so in effect burning the excess fat around your tummy. They strengthen and increase the power to your legs.

See 'Tip' for information on post-partum time.

Have your baby in the buggy or on a pillow or blanket.

Method for Tuck Jump

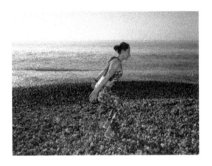

1. Have your feet slightly more than hip distance apart.

2. Bring your arms down by your hips, palms facing inwards. Drop the shoulders down away from your ears and engage your core

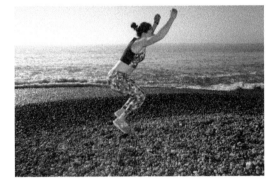

3. Have the knees slightly bent and engage your leg muscles. Drop the hips back and down so the tail bone is tucked under. Come into a half squat.

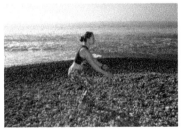

4. Using your arm muscles, propel upwards bending the knees in the air to tuck them up in towards the chest.

5. As you land, bend the knees slightly so the impact will not cause too much pressure in the joints.

Repeat as many times as you would like.

Method for Tuck Jump Using a Buggy

Follow the above instructions but hold onto the buggy handle having your arms on the handle width apart and extended. Bring your knees up but not right into your chest.

Tip

Be careful if your pelvic floor muscles are still healing. Pressure to this area may cause them to heal more slowly.

Be careful if you have a healing Diastasis Recti. This pose is not advisable if you still have quite a large gap.

If still healing then do not bring your knees up into your chest, go as far as is comfortable and work up towards this over the coming months.

If you are finding that you have urinary incontinence (I know, I have suffered with this too) due to the pelvic floor muscles still healing, then it's probably best not to do this exercise. The force when you land back on the floor is huge and this can set back any pelvic floor muscles you have built back up. Wait until around six months post-partum to do this exercise.

'Persistence is the most travelled path to success.' - Bryant Mcgill

Bow Pose

This pose has so many benefits. It is amazing at improving your posture. We tend to lose sight of our posture when carrying our children around. This pose strengthens all the muscles in the back, arms and shoulders and stretches out the chest, thighs, tops of feet and abdomen. It is an all-round great stretch. It also awakens the nerves in the spinal cord making your mind feel alive and energised. If you are feeling fatigued at all then this pose is great to wake you up.

Have your baby on a pillow or blanket next to you or in the buggy.

Method

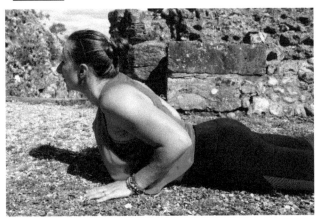

1. Come onto the floor on your tummy. Engage your gluteal muscles (buttocks) and bring your arms or hands either underneath your shoulders or palms down by your hips.

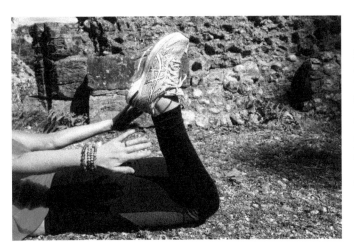

2. Bend your knees bringing the heels as close to your buttocks as possible and reach behind and grasp both ankles with your hands. Draw the shoulder blades backwards and towards the spine, keeping shoulders down away from your ears.

3. On your inhale lift through your chest, pushing your feet into your hands and opening through the chest creating a bow shape.

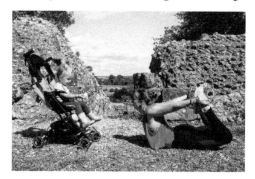 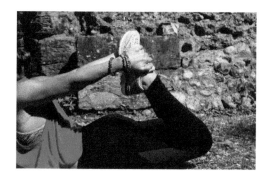

Keep your knees hip distance apart and try to draw the inner thighs inwards. Engage your quadriceps (quads) by lifting them off the floor while lifting the feet keeping shoulders back.

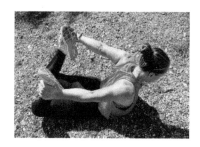

4. Breathe in this pose and with every exhale try to lift through the chest more.

5. Stay here for five to six breaths. Slowly come out and release back down to the floor, resting for as long as needed.

Tip

Be careful here if you have a serious lower back or neck injury.

If doing this outside, maybe lay on a mat or blanket.

If you cannot reach around to grasp your feet, then use a strap or resistance band to create extra length. Place it around the front of your ankles and grasp the band ends with both hands. You could also just reach round and grasp one ankle with your hand.

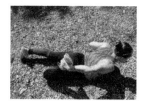

'Look for something positive in every day, Even if some days you have to look a little harder.' - Unknown

Page 188 Bow Pose

Kneeling Superman Exercise

This is a great way to stretch out the shoulders, strengthen the gluteal muscles (glutes) and work the core.

Have baby resting on a pillow in front of you or in the buggy.

Method

1. Come onto all fours, have your hands stacked under your shoulders spreading out your fingers and have knees hip width apart stacked under hips.

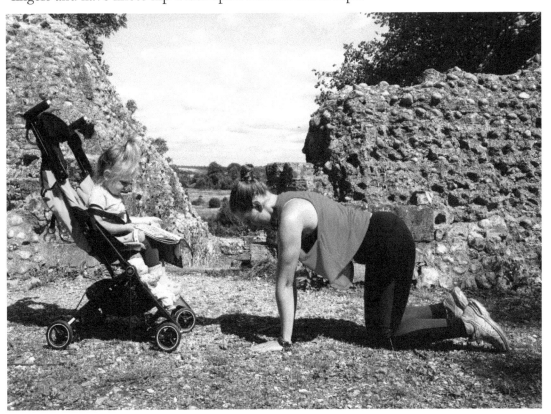

Push your shoulders away from the spine so as not to collapse in your chest.

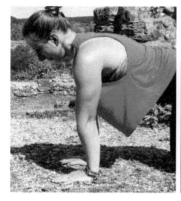 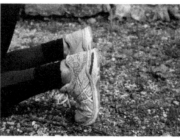 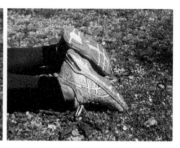

Toes can either be tucked under or pointing away.

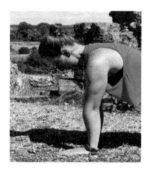

Have your gaze through to your hands and not further forwards or looking up as this will cause your neck and spine to be out of alignment. Tilt your chin slightly towards your chest, imagining holding a tennis ball there.

2. Engage your glutes, core and back, forming through your hands and lift the right arm up off the floor pointing it out in front of you. At the same time, lift the opposite leg out to the back, pushing heel away from you, pointing toes towards the floor. Aim to have them parallel to the floor.

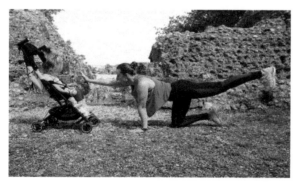

Heal pushed away, correct alignment.　Toes pushed away, not correct alignment.

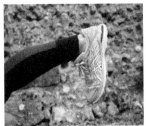

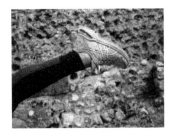

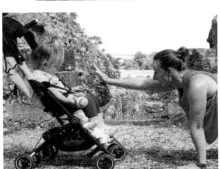

3. Try to keep the leg muscles engaged and reach through the middle finger. Push shoulders down away from the ears.

Hold for five breaths and slowly lower both limbs down to the start position.

4. Repeat five to ten times on each side.

Tip

Be careful in this exercise if you have knee problems. Place a cushion or blanket underneath to relieve any tension. If this is quite tight on your wrists, then hold onto the buggy footplate.

If new to doing Superman's, then repeat a couple of times to slowly build up the strength in the back and glutes.

Keep the elbows slightly bent and do not lock them out.

Breathe normally trying not to hold your breath.

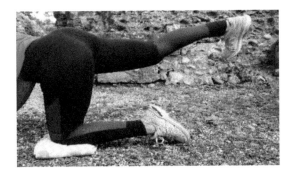

'I' is the only difference between FIT and FAT.'
– Goodlife fitness

Page 191 Kneeling Superman Exercise

Seated Spinal Twist

This is a real spinal twist and will squeeze your insides out, in a good way. This pose also stimulates the liver and kidneys and stretches the shoulders, hips, and neck. It energizes the spine and stimulates the digestive system. It relieves backache and it is therapeutic for asthma and infertility.

Have baby in a buggy or next to you on a comfy pillow or cushion for this pose.

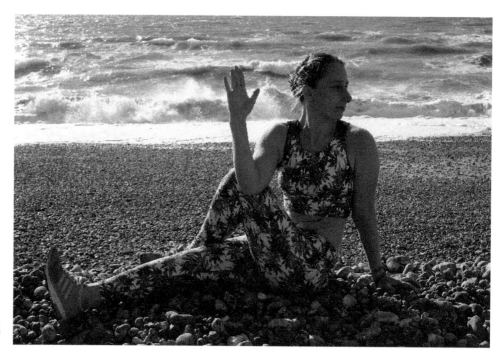

Method

1. Come onto the mat and come to a sitting position with your legs out in front of you. Come onto your sitting bones by pulling your buttocks away from you.

2. Bend the right leg over your left and place your right foot just the other side of your left knee resting on the floor.

3. Keeping the left leg straight, push the heel away from you, flexing the toes towards the shin engaging all the leg muscles.

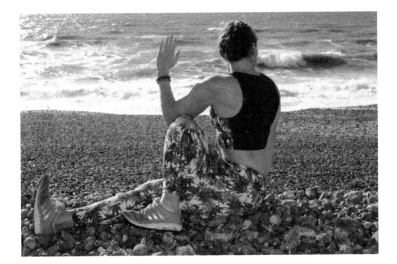

4. Bring your left elbow to rest on the middle or outside of your right knee with your hand pointing upwards, palm facing away from you.

5. With your right-hand place it behind you, pushing into the mat and twist round on your next exhale. If you are finding that your chest is collapsing here, use a block or a couple of rolled up towels or cushion to find that extra height.

6. On every inhale lift through the crown of your head and on every exhale twist the chest round further, making sure your torso is forward and up. Stay here for five breaths.

7. To come out of the pose, on your next inhale release your legs and swap to the other side.

Tip

Be aware in this pose if you have asthma or suffer with diarrhoea as the twist will help open the chest and open the bowels. Also, any issues with back pain or neck problems.

Be careful here if you have a healing Diastasis Recti. This pose is not advisable if you still have quite a large gap.

To advance this you can bind it if you wish. Bring your right armpit over your right knee and bend your right arm around the side of your thigh. With your left arm, bring it behind you on your left side. Back of hand facing towards the spine. Try and clasp your hands. Look up and twist around over your left shoulder. Swap sides.

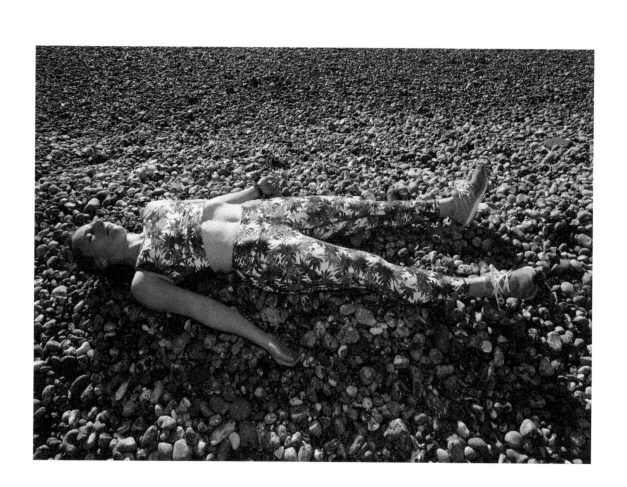

Chapter Seven

Meditation and Relaxation Guide

Meditation and Relaxation Guide

As parents we all need to relax at some point in our day. We need to try to set aside some time, even if it's just five minutes each day. You can do it before your household wakes up, or while the children are playing or once they've gone to bed. This will really help your mind, concentration and overall general health and well-being.

This relaxation technique will also help with post-natal depression. If you feel like you are not coping with life or parenting, try this technique. Gather all your thoughts, put them in a bubble and blow them away with your exhale. Say to yourself, 'relax, refresh, recharge'.

One of my favourite quotes from Bryant Mcgill is, 'Your calm mind is the ultimate weapon against your challenges. So, relax.' To me this sums up parenting challenges. You need a calm mind to see through and past the challenges we face every day, especially if you are sleep deprived in the early months of parenthood.

Method

Come to a seated or laying down position.

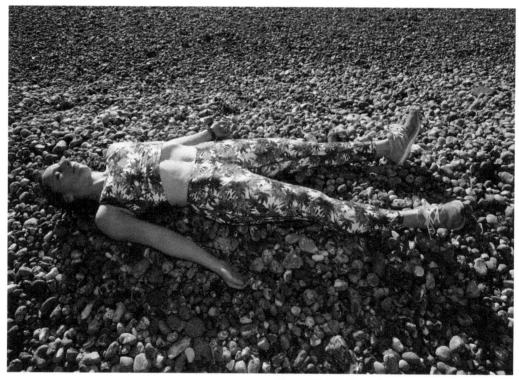

If seated, get comfortable and have hands resting wherever is comfortable. If laying down, have your feet more than hip distance apart, hands down by your sides slightly away from your chest, having the palms facing towards the sky. Gently push your shoulders down away from your ears and tilt your head so your chin is slightly facing towards the chest. This will lengthen the spine. Gently close your eyes and bring the tongue away from the roof of your mouth. Have your jaw slightly open, releasing tension in your face. Move any part of your body you need to, to feel comfortable. You need to fully release all the muscles. Fully release all the thoughts. Fully release all the tension kept in your body. Have a wriggle, have a giggle, and then settle down to your final comfortable relaxation state.

Slowly start to gather your thoughts, collecting them all up and putting them in a bubble and blowing them away with your exhale. Any other thoughts that come your way, let them go. Let them just drift past, trying not to cling onto them. You want your mind and body to be completely still.

Be conscious of your breathing for three deep breaths. Inhale using your diaphragm. Try breathing from the bottom of your tummy right up to the top of your collar bone. You are aiming to fully inflate your lungs. Gently push your shoulder blades down into the floor, spreading them away from your ears and away from the spine. On every inhale slightly pause at the top before your exhale. Do not pause if you have high blood pressure.

On your exhales you are aiming to slowly release from the tops of your collar bone, down through the chest, using your core muscles to push out all the extra air. Slowly count to three on the inhales and four on the exhales. On the inhale say to yourself, 'let' and on your exhales say to yourself, 'go'. Listen to your body and feel it releasing. Releasing tension all over your body.

Find your final relaxation state. Notice your breath's natural rhythm, allowing the tummy to rise and fall naturally.

Starting at the tips of your toes and working all the way to the crown of the head, relax all the muscles and bones in your body. Imagine the muscles peeling away from the bones. Relaxing.

Slowly relaxing the soles of the feet, ankles, calves and shins. Relax the knees, kneecaps, back of knees. Relax your thighs (quads and hamstrings). Bring your attention towards the front of your pelvis and start to relax. Relax the hip joints, the front and back of the pelvis. The top and bottom of the pelvis. There is so much tension kept in the pelvis area. Breathe into the area deeply. Relax the lower spine, feeling the back muscles peeling away from it. Bring your attention around to the front of your body. Relax your internal organs, your tummy area. Relax the middle of your spine, chest ribs, the muscles in between the ribs (intercostal muscles). Relax the top of your spine. The collar bones. Bring your attention to the shoulder blades. Relax the shoulders. Relax your upper arms (triceps and biceps). Relax your elbows, forearms, wrists, hands and fingers. Imagine someone lifting your arm up and releasing it to the floor. It would be so heavy that it would fall quickly. Bring your attention towards the back of the neck, relaxing the muscles. The front of the neck, relaxing the thyroid glands, voice box. Relax your head. Feeling your head heavy, sinking into the floor. Bring your attention to your face. Relax your forehead, eyes, cheek bones, jaw. Finally relaxing your mind.

Stay here for as long as you need to. Breathing in and out. Clearing your mind.

Visualisation – When fully relaxed, slowly start to visualise yourself marooned on a deserted beach. No one else around but you. Sitting under a palm tree gazing out to the crystal-clear waters of the ocean. Imagine the colours around you. Bright blue sky, green palm tree leaves, white soft sand. Imagine picking up the nice white soft sand and letting it run through your fingers and toes. Noticing how soft and pure it feels. Noticing the gentle breeze on your skin, the warm sun beaming down on you. Letting all your thoughts and worries go. Listening to the waves gently lapping on the shore. Just feeling calm, relaxed, being present in this present moment.

You may want to take a walk down to the ocean. Slowly get up from where you are sitting under your palm tree. Walk down to the ocean feeling the soft white sand between your toes. Feeling the warm sun still beaming down on you. Maybe picking up some shells as you go. As you reach the shoreline, slowly take a paddle into the shallow water. Noticing the coolness of the ocean around your feet and ankles. Watching little fish swim around your feet. Feeling your feet sinking into the sand. Maybe stay here or take a walk through the water. Just walking gently. Noticing your feelings.

How calm, relaxed, and heavy the body feels. Stay here for as long or as little as you wish. Start to slowly walk back up the beach, feeling the soft sand around your toes. Gently sit back down under your palm tree. Still gazing out to the ocean. Noticing how calm and relaxed you are.

As you slowly start to bring your mind back into the room, gently wriggling your fingers and toes bringing the sensation back into your body. Maybe hug your knees into your chest or have a stretch and a yawn. Bring the right arm up above your head and slowly, when you are ready, roll onto your right side, resting your head on your arm. Stay here for as long as you wish. Noticing how relaxed, calm, and heavy your body feels. When you are ready, push up to a comfortable seated position, hands resting wherever is comfortable.

We are going to take three long, big deep breaths. Slowly inhale and slowly exhale. On the second breath inhale to fully expand your lungs, pausing at the top only if this is comfortable and then on the exhale really releasing any tension held here. On your last breath, take a big deep inhale using all your lung capacity and a bit more. On your exhale let out a big sigh. Noticing how your body feels after your relaxation and breathing.

You are now free to carry on with your day, or if practicing this at night, rest soundly feeling calm, relaxed, and rested.

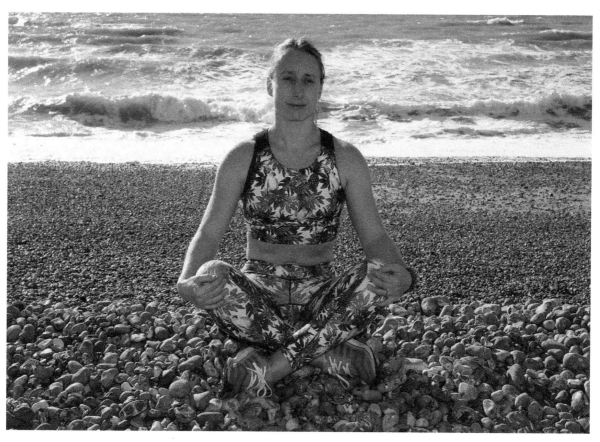

Figure 4 - Cross Legged Seated Pose

Here sleeps a girl with a heart full of magical dreams,

A heart full of wonder,

And hands that will shape the world.' –
Thesayingquotes.com

Chapter Eight

Four-week Yoga
Exercise Training
Programme

Four-week Yoga Exercise Training Programme

Here is a four-week easy to follow programme created for you to get back to your fitness or to find your fitness after becoming a parent. This will follow a pattern from easy poses to getting harder each week. It will include a variety of strength and relaxing yoga poses burning fat, building muscles, building strength in the core muscles, and generally getting you moving. It will also help to stretch and lengthen the muscles in the body.

Follow the plan and you will notice how much stronger and fitter you will feel. Follow a good balanced diet in line with this programme and see the results. You can also make up your own version using the poses and exercises in this book.

The equipment you will need will be:

- Baby wrap/sling
- Park bench
- Tree or vertical wall
- Buggy
- Yoga mat, but not essential

Repeat each set for the stated number of reps or for the more advanced, up your reps in each set. Have fun, enjoy and good luck.

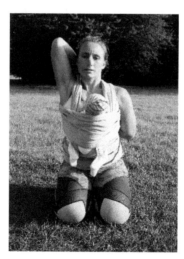

WEEK ONE

	WARM UP	DAY ONE	DAY TWO	DAY THREE	DAY FOUR	DAY FIVE	DAY SIX	DAY SEVEN
WEEK ONE	Warm up each day - Gentle five minute walk.	Head and Neck Stretches	Rest day or a gentle walk	Mountain Pose	Rest day or gentle walk	Standing Side Bend and Back Bend	Rest day or gentle walk	Cat and Cow Pose
	Throughout the workout staying in each pose for one to two minutes.	Standing Side Bends and Back Bends		Cat and Cow Pose		Step-ups step-up side kick x5-10 on each leg		Slow Sun Salutation A
	Repeating each set three times.	Half Forward Fold		Butterfly Pose		Bridge Pose		Seated Spinal Twist

	WARM UP	DAY ONE	DAY TWO	DAY THREE	DAY FOUR	DAY FIVE	DAY SIX	DAY SEVEN
WEEK TWO	Warm up each day - Gentle five minute walk.	Sun Salutation A	Rest or a gentle walk.	Lunges baby wrap or buggy x 5-10 on each leg	Rest or a gentle walk	Boat Pose	Rest day or a gentle walk	Head and neck stretch
	Throughout workout staying in each pose for one to two minutes	Tree Pose		Triangle Pose using buggy		Camel Pose		Plank and Plank Advances
	Repeating each set three times.	Side Angle Stretch pushing buggy		Calf raises and calf raise walks x10 on each leg		Cow Face Pose		Warrior Two + pushing buggy

	WARM UP	DAY ONE	DAY TWO	DAY THREE	DAY FOUR	DAY FIVE	DAY SIX	DAY SEVEN
WEEK THREE	Warm up each day - Gentle five-minute walk or slowly building up to a gentle jog or run.	Head and neck stretch	Rest or a ten-minute walk, jog or run	Tricep dips x10	Rest or a ten to fifteen-minute walk, jog or run.	Step-ups step-up side kick x10	Rest or a 10 to 15-minute walk, jog or run.	Tree Pose with or without baby
	Throughout the workout staying in each pose for one to two minutes.	Cat and Cow Pose. Wall sit. Sun Salutation B.		Chest Press with baby. Cow Face Pose.		Camel Pose. Burpees (as many as you can do in 1 minute)		Squat and walking squat with buggy. Dancer holding onto buggy
	Repeating each set three times. Staying in the poses or flows for a little longer. Try to push past your comfort zone. This week we will be doing four or five poses.	Warrior Three push outs using buggy		Downward Dog to Plank x10. Tuck Jumps x8		Kneeling Superman's. Side Angle Stretch pushing buggy		Calf raises and calf raise walks. Chair Pose

WARM UP	DAY ONE	DAY TWO	DAY THREE	DAY FOUR	DAY FIVE	DAY SIX	DAY SEVEN
	Warm up each day - Gentle 10-minute walk, jog or run.	Camel Pose	Kneeling Superman's		Downward Dog to Plank walkouts x6	Warrior Three push outs using buggy	Cat and Cow Pose
WEEK FOUR	Throughout the workout staying in each pose for one to two minutes. Repeating each set four times. Keep going you are doing so well. We are nearly there.	Tree Pose and Triangle Pose	Wall Sit	Rest Day or a gentle walk	Triangle Pose	Tree Pose	Warrior 2
		Chest Press or Push-up variations x6	Dancer Pose		Hand to Knee Pose or Hand to Toe Pose	Dancer Pose	Head and Neck Stretches
		Burpees (as many as you can do in 1 minute)	Tuck Jumps x10 Bridge Pose		Tricep Dips x10 Boat V-Sit	Burpees (as many as you can do in 1 minute)	Tuck Jumps x10 Bridge Pose

Index

References

Pelvic floor references

www.popg.csp.org.uk The Pelvic Floor Muscles Guide For Women
POGP Administration Fitwise Management Ltd, Blackburn House, Redhouse Road,
Seafield, Bathgate, West Lothian, EH47 7AQ
Date accessed 06/11/2018

www.nhs.uk
What are pelvic floor exercises
Date accessed 06/11/2018

Diastasis Recti References

www.parents.com
Parents.com is part of the Parents Network. © Copyright 2019 Meredith Corporation
Date accessed 12/10/2018

www.babycentre.com
BabyCenter, L.L.C. 1997-2019
By Amy Paturel
Reviewed by the BabyCenter Medical Advisory Board
January 31, 2017
Date accessed 12/10/2018

www.nhs.uk - Your post pregnancy body.
Date accessed 12/10/2018

Nutrition References

British Nutrition Foundation 2018. www.nutrition.org.uk - Protein, Fats and Carbohydrates
Date accessed 08/08/2018

2005 - 2019 WebMD LLC
www.webmd.com - Protein
Date accessed 17/08/2018

British Heart Foundation Greater London House, 180 Hampstead Road, London NW1
7AW.
www.bhf.org.uk - Protein
Date accessed 08/080/2018

BSY Yoga Teacher (Hatha Yoga) Qualification Level Four Award.
Subject Nutrition Unit 8 and 9
Date qualification gained 29th August 2013
Principle Ann Williams

www.nhs.uk - Nutrition Overview Eat Well
Date accessed 25/09/2018

www.livestrong.com Partner and Licensee of the Livestrong Foundation. Leaf Group Ltd.
Date accessed 19/09/2018

www.livescience.com - Carbohydrates
Live Science is part of Future US Inc, an international media group
Future US, Inc. 11 West 42nd Street, 15th Floor, New York, NY 10036.

<u>Instagram posts for inspiration</u>
@Danwheeler<u>8020</u> Daniel Wheeler
@bwmcfitness Jennifer Gelman PhD
@kayla_itsines Kayla Itsines
@fitmomma4three Melanie Darnell

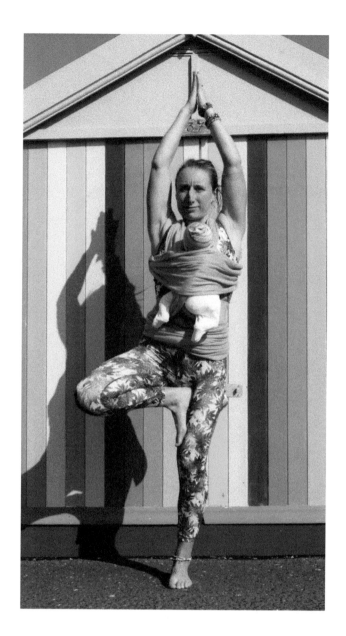

CONTACT DETAILS

If you are in need of a little motivation or inspiration or would like some more tips and advice then go to www.easyoga.co.uk to see videos, articles, blog posts and more. If you have any questions or comments, then please do not hesitate to get in touch:

www.easyoga.co.uk

www.easyoga.co.uk/easyogablog

gemmanice82@gmail.com

Facebook: Gemma Nice

Facebook Page: www.facebook.com/EasYogaOnet oOne

Twitter: @yogigemma

Instagram: @yogigemma

Pintrest: Yogigemma

YouTube: Easyoga Gemma

LinkedIn: https://www.linkedin.com/in/%F 0%9F%A7%98%E2%80%8D%E 2%99%80%EF%B8%8Fgemma-nice-97a52819a/

Lightning Source UK Ltd.
Milton Keynes UK
UKHW050655141220
375035UK00003B/27